Solution Focused Coaching Supervision

Solution Focused Coaching Supervision offers the reader a theoretically coherent framework for coaching supervision, outlined in an engaging way that is simple to understand and apply immediately using a variety of collaborative coaching supervision moves grounded in practical examples.

The book offers an in-depth understanding of the theory of Solution Focused (SF) Supervision, which, as a social-constructionist approach, privileges the coaching supervision clients' experience, resources and preferred future over an "analytic" or deficit-oriented stance. It also provides a step-by-step "how-to" for individual, group, peer and team coaching supervision. Coaching supervision ethics is discussed in theory and via real-case examples. Deliberate and reflective practice models will enable readers to develop their practice wherever their starting point may be. The reader will also find transcripts of actual coaching supervision sessions to bring the theory to life.

An essential and comprehensive resource that will enable beginner coaching supervisors to start practising this highly respectful and ethical approach to coaching supervision, while also inspiring more advanced coaching supervisors to use this simple and effective approach to coaching supervision.

Kirsten Dierolf is the owner and founder of Solutions Academy, an International Coaching Federation (ICF)– and European Mentoring and Coaching Council (EMCC)–accredited coach training school. Kirsten started her journey with the SF approach when she studied directly with its founders, Insoo Kim Berg and Steve de Shazer and since then has been passionate about the SF and other social-constructionist approaches. She has been supervising coaches since 2006 and training coaching supervisors since 2022.

Svea van der Hoorn is an accredited coach, educational psychologist, accredited coaching supervisor, mentor coach, educator and author. She discovered the SF approach in 1989, and it continues to infuse her work. Svea has experience with the diversity of supervision frameworks and practices, having supervised teachers, psychologists, SF therapists and coaches, individually and in groups, since 1985.

Debbie Hogan is the founder and owner of the Academy of Solution Focused Training and was the first to bring SF coaching and SF certification to Asia. Her coach training is accredited by the ICF for Associate Certified Coach, Professional Certified Coach, and Master Certified Coach. She was deeply impacted when she trained with Insoo Kim Berg and Steve de Shazer in their inaugural Graduate Diploma in SF Brief Therapy. Debbie has been a trainer and supervisor for more than 30 years, working with individuals, groups and teams and with supervisors seeking certification.

Jane Tuomola is an accredited coach, clinical psychologist, accredited coaching supervisor, trainer and author. She was introduced to the SF approach in 2009 and uses this in all areas of her work. She has a particular passion for developing others through supervision and has been supervising since 2006 and training supervisors since 2014.

"*Social Focused Coaching Supervision* offers the opportunity for supervisors to further extend their practice through a social constructionist, collaborative, Solution Focused approach to coaching supervision. Skilfully written, practically focussed and insightful, Dierolf and her colleagues offer the reader both an opportunity to deepen their understanding and apply this evidenced based approach to their practice."

Professor Jonathan Passmore, *Henley Business School, UK*

"*Solution Focused Coaching Supervision* provides a unique perspective on coaching supervision grounded in a social constructionist paradigm which has much to offer coaching practice. The book is practical, informative and beneficial for supervisors, coaches and educators."

Dr. Adrian Myers, *MA Coaching and Mentoring,*
Oxford Brookes University, UK

"This book provides food for thought for all professional supervisors and those planning to train in supervision. In particular, reflective practice will take on increasing importance in our professions."

Dr. Michel Moral, *MSc, PhD, Cergy-Pontoise University, France*

"This book is most timely as it offers a new perspective on developmental Supervision in coaching. It is perfectly balanced in its structure and clear in its content. If you are serious about Supervision in coaching, this is a must read."

Professor Bob Garvey, *Leeds Business School, UK*

"This is a welcome addition to the literature on Coaching Supervision. It's a great resource that will enable coaches and supervisors to find the best support for themselves and to explore different approaches that will add to their knowledge and CPD. It offers a detailed description of *Solution Focused Coaching Supervision* for both individuals and groups. It includes case studies to bring the subject to life. This book will help to raise the global profile of Supervision."

Carol Whitaker, *Oxford Brookes University, UK*

"Even a quick mention of the word "supervision" anywhere in the coaching world gets a strong reaction. Some coaches love supervision. Some coaches see it as a box to check on the way to a credential. And still other coaches find supervision to be something they're just trying out. Bottom line from my experience: Coaches who are committed to supervision demonstrate that they are serious about their craft and their professional development.

What Kirsten Dierolf and colleagues have done in this work is keep the focus on supporting coaches by leveraging the supervision process. Whether it's exploring a change model, client growth, supervision strategy or the ethics of coaching supervision, this book will sharpen your supervision skills and by extension, your coaching."

Jonathan Reitz, *MCC, ACTC, Case Western Reserve University, USA*

"This book about coaching supervision from a social constructionist/ Solution Focused perspective is an instant classic. Whether you are a professional supervisor or starting to become engaged with others, this book gives you a myriad ways to take an open and enabling stance to supervise ethically, encouragingly and professionally."

Dr. Mark McKergow, *Author of* The Next Generation of Solution Focused Practice

"As readers journey through this book, they can look out for a golden thread weaving through each element of the authors' supervision practice – the solution focused approach. This clear methodological perspective provides an internally consistent reference point for decision-making, ethics and best practice. A distinct addition to the developing field of coaching supervision"

Jo Birch, Supervisor, *Executive Coach, Psychotherapist, Author and Editor*

Solution Focused Coaching Supervision

An Essential Guide for Individual, Group, Peer and Team Coaching Supervision

**Edited by Kirsten Dierolf,
Svea van der Hoorn,
Debbie Hogan and
Jane Tuomola**

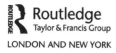

Routledge
Taylor & Francis Group

LONDON AND NEW YORK

Designed cover image: Copyright [Boris Znaev]/Adobe Stock

First published 2025
by Routledge
4 Park Square, Milton Park, Abingdon, Oxon OX14 4RN

and by Routledge
605 Third Avenue, New York, NY 10158

*Routledge is an imprint of the Taylor & Francis Group,
an informa business*

© 2025 selection and editorial matter, Kirsten Dierolf, Svea van der Hoorn, Debbie Hogan and Jane Tuomola; individual chapters, the contributors

British Library Cataloguing-in-Publication Data
A catalogue record for this book is available from the British Library

Library of Congress Cataloging-in-Publication Data
Names: Dierolf, Kirsten, editor. | Van der Hoorn, Svea, editor. | Hogan, Debbie, editor. | Tuomola, Jane, editor.
Title: Solution focused coaching supervision : an essential guide for individual, group, peer and team coaching supervision / edited by Kirsten Dierolf, Svea van der Hoorn, Debbie Hogan and Jane Tuomola.
Description: Abingdon, Oxon ; New York, NY : Routledge, 2025. | Includes bibliographical references and index.
Identifiers: LCCN 2024013557 | ISBN 9781032487397 (hardback) | ISBN 9781032487380 (paperback) | ISBN 9781003390527 (ebook)
Subjects: LCSH: Supervision. | Solution-focused therapy. | Personal coaching. | Executive coaching.
Classification: LCC HM1253 .S65 2025 |
DDC 658.3/124--dc23/eng/20240614
LC record available at https://lccn.loc.gov/2024013557

ISBN: 9781032487397 (hbk)
ISBN: 9781032487380 (pbk)
ISBN: 9781003390527 (ebk)

DOI: 10.4324/9781003390527

Typeset in Galliard
by KnowledgeWorks Global Ltd.

Contents

Biographies of the Editors

Kirsten Dierolf, MA, MSFP, ICF MCC, EMCC MP, EMCC ESIA, EMCC ITCA MP, Kirsten has been coaching executives, middle managers and teams for global corporations since 1996 and for over 3000 hours. She also designed and delivered large leadership development programmes all over the globe. In 2016 she was certified as Master Certified Coach and as EMCC Master Practitioner. She holds EMCC and ICF team coaching accreditation and is an accredited coach supervisor with EMCC. Kirsten is a member of the assessor team for the ICF for MCC and PCC credentials as well as a trained assessor for EMCC. Kirsten is the owner and founder of "SolutionsAcademy", a coach training institute accredited by ICF and EMCC which has been teaching coaching in online programmes since 2008. The main focus of SolutionsAcademy is social-constructionist approaches like SF and Narrative Practice. Kirsten's SF expertise comes from training directly with the founders of the approach, Insoo Kim Berg and Steve de Shazer. She was president of SFCT, the association for the quality development of SF consulting and training and founder and member of the editorial team for *InterAction—The Journal of Solution Focus in Organisations*. She studied Narrative Practices at the Dulwich Center in Adelaide, Australia. She has been a coaching supervisor since 2006 and training coaching supervisors since 2022. She is a prolific writer with over 40 articles and 3 books: *The Solution Tango* with Louis Cauffman, and *Solution Focused Team Coaching* and *Becoming a Master Coach*.

Svea van der Hoorn, DEd (Ed Psych), ICF MCC, EMCC SP, EMCC ESIA, discovered the SF approach in 1989 while looking for resources for postgraduate students in educational psychology, computer science and engineering management, who were exploring constructive conversations. She has never stopped reading about, reflecting on, imagining and applying the SF principles and practices in her work, whether that be adult education, supervision, ICF mentor coaching for credentialing purposes, end-of-life-as-you-know-it coaching, leadership and decision-making coaching or writing support. Svea is a self-declared ethics nerd. She loves the creativity that emerges from engaging with complexity, ambiguity and uncertainty. She volunteers on the ICF Independent Review Board (ICF IRB), contributing to resolving ethical complaints lodged against individual ICF professionals. She keeps herself aware of coaches' experiences by volunteering in professional associations as a subject matter expert. Svea's background in mental health, family and individual therapy was gained working in socio-economic and political contexts characterised by hardship, unfair discrimination and poor governance. She remains a pragmatic optimist and keeps ingenuity alive in adverse circumstances. She has contributed to Solutions Academy since its inception. She has contributed chapters to a number of SF and/or coaching books.

Debbie Hogan, MS, MSFP, ICF MCC, EMCC MP, EMCC ESIA, is the founder and Managing Director of the Academy of Solution Focused Training Pte Ltd. Since 2004, she and her team of associates have been involved in the quality development of training SF practitioners across the globe and supporting this growing community in Asia and beyond. She trained with Insoo Kim Berg and Steve de Shazer, the developers of SF practice in 1999 and earned the first Graduate Diploma in SF Brief Therapy. In Private Practice since 1993 as a psychotherapist, she works within a wide spectrum of clinical issues, as an Executive and Leadership Coach with teams and individuals, and as a supervisor and mentor coach. She is a Master Clinical Member and Clinical Supervisor with the Singapore Association for Counseling. Debbie is a founding member of International Alliance of Solution Focused Teaching Institutes, Master Certified Coach with the ICF, Master Practitioner and Accredited Coach Supervisor with the EMCC. Her coach training is accredited with the ICF at Level 1 ACC, Level 2 PCC and Level 3 MCC. Debbie has edited and contributed to four books, including *Solution Focused Practice in Asia* with Dave Hogan, Jane Tuomola and Alan Yeo and *Solution Focused Practice Around the World* with Kirsten Dierolf, Sukanya Wignaraja and Svea van der Hoorn. She is co-editor of SF Coaching in Asia with Jane Tuomola and Sukanya Wignarja, to be published in 2024.

Jane Tuomola, DClinPsy, MSFP, ICF PCC, EMCC SP, EMCC ESIA, has her own company in Singapore where she has worked for 11 years. She works as both a Clinical Psychologist (specialising in adult mental health) and as a Life and Executive Coach, and Coaching Supervisor. She is an Associate Fellow of the British Psychological Society and Master Solution Focused Practitioner with the International Alliance of Solution Focused Teaching Institutes. As a coach, she is a Professional Certified Coach with the ICF and a Senior Practitioner with the EMCC. Jane's particular area of expertise is supervision. She has over 16 years of experience as a clinical supervisor and 6 years of experience as a coaching supervisor. She offers both individual and group supervisions, as well as teaching SF supervision to therapists and coaches. She is an approved supervisor with the Canadian Council of Professional Certification and an accredited coach supervisor with the EMCC. She is an Associate Trainer and Supervisor with the Academy of Solution Focused Training in Singapore and SolutionsAcademy in Germany. She is a co-editor of two books: *Solution Focused Practice in Asia and Solution Focused Coaching in Asia* and also has written research articles and other book chapters.

Biographies of the Authors

Chris Bekker, ICF-PCC, EMCC-SP, EMCC-ESIA, Chris is a certified coach and coaching supervisor. He had an eclectic start to his professional life: travelling the world and working at every job he could find, from bartending in Australia to anti-poaching in South Africa. He started working as an English teacher in Johannesburg and subsequently took up job offers in Somalia, Kenya, Russia and Ukraine, as a teacher, consultant and eventually a coach. While seeking certified coach training he found SolutionsAcademy where he discovered the fascinating world of SF and narrative approaches in coaching and has been blessed to be a part of the team at SolutionsAcademy for the past five years. Amongst his clients, he has worked with TV personalities, professional footballers, TED speakers, business owners, negotiators, lawyers and anyone who finds benefit from taking time out to think about and reflect on their path. Chris divides his time between training coaches, mentoring those coaches, supervising coaches who are looking for thinking space or other support and partaking in the adventures that make life a richer learning experience. He currently lives in Sardinia with his best friend, wife and partner Fede.

Cristina Mühl, ICF-PCC, ICF-ACTC, EMCC-SP, EMCC-ITCA SP, EMCC-IPMA, EMCC-ESIA, is an accredited coach and team coach both with ICF and EMCC and also an accredited supervisor, working with team coaches to develop their own practice. She started coaching using the SF approach in 2019 and since then moved also into delivering training based on the approach. Cristina studied with Kirsten and is now humbled to be part of the further development of SolutionsAcademy internationally and locally in Romania. Her contributions to the evolution of coaching extend beyond her individual practice. She has been involved in several initiatives such as EMCC Global Research Group, EMCC Global Upskilling Group, Subject Matter Expert with ICF Global on coaching supervision, demonstrating her leadership and vision for the future of coaching in her region. Furthermore, Cristina has contributed to the knowledge base of coaching with the published book on team coaching – *Solution Focused Team Coaching* in collaboration with Kirsten Dierolf, Carlo Perfetto and Rafal Szaniawski.

Carlo Perfetto, ICF-PCC, EMCC-SP, EMCC-ESIA, has been a very passionate trainer for almost 25 years on soft skills, leadership and communication in business environments. He has always worked with medium-high management levels in leading corporations. He has also had two experiences in multinational companies as a Training and Development Manager, but he has always returned to his primary passion: training. In 2013 he started to study and apply the SF approach to the training programmes he has developed over the years and in the coaching teams in which he took part as a facilitator. At the same time, he also focused on supporting others in their personal and professional development in a more "personalised" form through coaching. In 2018 he became a PCC with SolutionsAcademy with which he currently collaborates as coach trainer, mentor and supervisor for the support of those who want to access the ACC and PCC accreditation levels. In the meantime, he is happily making his way to becoming MCC.

Sukanya Wignaraja, MSc/DipSW (Oxon), ICF-PCC, EMCC-SP, EMCC-ESIA, has a Masters in Social Work from Oxford University, UK. She is a Master Solution Focused Practitioner with the International Alliance of Solution Focused Teaching Institutes and a Professional Certified Coach with the International Coach Federation. Sukanya worked in the mental health field in the UK for many years across a range of settings, including community teams, hospitals and the prison service. She was a Specialist Advisor in Social Work to the UK Foreign & Commonwealth Office. Sukanya was an Executive Coach and Senior Psychotherapist in mental health NGOs in Manila and Tokyo, where she also conducted training programmes for counsellors. Since 2017, Sukanya has been in private practice in Colombo, Sri Lanka where she works with individuals and couples and as an Executive Coach. Sukanya is a Mentor Coach and Associate Coach Trainer with the Academy of Solution Focused Training. She is a Clinical Supervisor and is Co-Director of the Academy's Peer Supervision Programme. Sukanya was co-editor of *Solution Focused Practice Around the World* with Kiersten Dierolf, Debbie Hogan and Svea van der Hoorn and is co-editor of the forthcoming *Solution Focused Coaching in Asia* with Debbie Hogan and Jane Tuomola.

Acknowledgements

This book is for the participants of our supervision classes and our supervision clients from whom we have learned so much: Thank you!

Kirsten Dierolf

As a supervisor, I draw from the wisdom of everyone who invited me to grow into the human being and supervisor that I am: my friends, colleagues, therapists, coaches and supervisors. This book would have never happened without their love and compassion and gentle nudges towards growth: thank you!

Svea van der Hoorn

Each supervision session reminds me of what I have forgotten, what I have not yet encountered and what is familiar. It is a wonderful university of life that continues to invite me to live with an awareness of opportunity and possibility. It is also a landscape in which I experience how words make worlds, often despite the factual circumstances.

Debbie Hogan

As I reflect on all the people who have impacted me in the supervision space, I'm profoundly grateful. Personally touched by so many who shared their challenges, struggles and desires to be better at their craft. I dedicate this book to the best partner one could have in life and work, Dave and to my incredibly gifted daughter, Breda and her husband, Joel, who just amaze me. Their love and never-ending support during the writing of this book I cherish so much. And to Kirsten, Svea and Jane, thank you for sharing this journey with me.

Jane Tuomola

This book is dedicated to Katharine Boon – my first supervisor. Thank you for supporting me as a very anxious first-year Clinical Psychology trainee. I was inspired to become a supervisor because of you. Thank you to Debbie, Kirsten and Svea for your part as trainers, supervisors and mentors in my coaching journey – it has been an honour to work with you on this project. Thank you to my husband Petri for supporting me during the writing and editing process – I couldn't have done it without you. And to my children who will finally get mummy back fully present in their lives – thanks for your patience and helping me laugh along the way!

Foreword

Coaching supervision is a relatively new professional development activity that supports the development of the coach, in service of their clients and the wider system. It has been part of the coaching scene in Europe for over 20 years and started to emerge in other parts of the world, such as North America, about 15 years ago.

Supervision originates from other helping professions such as therapy and counselling. There is a conversation emerging on whether it is time for coaching supervision to claim its own space apart from the therapeutic world. What differentiates coaching supervision from other supervision spaces? This will be an interesting discussion to engage in as the concept of supervision is introduced into other professions, such as leadership and facilitation.

This book, *Solution Focused Coaching Supervision*, invites a SF approach to coaching supervision. This way mostly looks at enhancing and doing more of what has been working to date, and less focus on the psychodynamics of the human psyche. As coaching supervision claims its space, this is one of many approaches to coaching supervision. The editors Kirsten Dierolf, Svea van de Hoorn, Debbie Hogan and Jane Tuomola along with authors Chris Bekker, Cristina Mühl, Carlo Perfetto and Sukanya Wignaraja explore important topics, including what SF coaching supervision is, ethical considerations, acknowledging different coaching models and the intersect between coaching supervision and mentoring and mentor coaching. Readers will also appreciate real examples of individual, group and peer SF coaching supervision, and how to supervise team coaches. The other point to note is that the authors look at the topic through the lens of the two largest coaching associations, the ICF and the EMCC.

This is one of the first books to deliberately engage in the conversation about differentiating coaching supervision from other supervision spaces. Kudos to the authors for stepping into this space.

Lily Seto, MA, PCC, ESIA, Master Practitioner
Co-host of the Americas (and Beyond)
Coaching Supervision Network

1 Introduction

Kirsten Dierolf and Svea van der Hoorn

Why This Book and Why Now?

Coaching supervision is a hot topic in coaching circles. The major coaching credentialing agencies, Association for Coaching (AC), European Mentoring and Coaching Council (EMCC) and International Coaching Federation (ICF), require coaches to undertake coaching supervision for various certifications. There is a growing need for coaching supervisors, as ICF has just begun to require 10 hours coaching supervision for gaining the "Advanced Certificate in Team Coaching", AC requires supervision for accreditation and EMCC requires accredited coaches to take at least 1 hour of coaching supervision per quarter or per 35 coaching sessions they deliver. The credentialing agencies have also recognised the need for professionalisation of coaching supervisors: ICF requires coaching supervisors to have a training of at least 60 hours. EMCC and AC offer an accreditation for coaching supervisors: the European Supervision Individual Accreditation (ESIA) for EMCC and Accredited Coach Supervisor for AC. All of these developments are recent, some starting as late as 2020.

Requiring supervision is typical of serious helping professions like psychotherapy or social work. As a young profession, coaching is looking to be taken as seriously. Maybe this is another reason for the growing interest in coaching supervision, apart from the obvious usefulness of an individual, customised learning path for practitioners of complex professions. It is understandable that coaches and coach educators might look to best practice or what's tried and tested in established supervision in allied professions to build the definition of, requirements for and methods to be used in coaching supervision. However, we propose that this is to miss the opportunity to establish coaching supervision as being isomorphic with and responsive to professional coaching, rather than with allied professions.

Given the growing market for coaching supervision, there will be an increasing interest in learning about coaching supervision, and a commensurate growing demand for skilled and accredited coaching supervisors. We are certainly becoming aware of a heightened interest in and registration for our EMCC-accredited coaching supervision courses.

DOI: 10.4324/9781003390527-1

If you are interested in either participating in or providing coaching supervision, this book will be a value-adding resource. While there are books on supervision in the helping professions, there are only a few books that address coaching supervision. For those who are already accomplished supervisors who wish to expand into coaching supervision, this book can offer the equivalent of a bridging course.

To date, there is no book that offers insights into Solution Focused coaching supervision and this book aspires to fill this gap. In this book, you will learn about coaching supervision with a consistent philosophical framework: a social constructionist, collaborative, Solution Focused approach to coaching supervision. Solution Focused coaching supervision pays attention to the coaching supervision client's growth and resources. It is less interested in explaining the past or the individual psyche of the coaching supervision client. It is totally not interested in generating any theories about the coaching supervision client's coaching client. Solution Focused coaching supervision works with the coaching supervisor and the coaching supervision client as the relevant system. Now for some glimpses into what the chapters offer you.

Overview of Chapters

Chapter 2 offers you an overview of the field of coaching supervision to date. It provides a short history of supervision in general and describes several strands of its origin as well as a history of the recent developments towards coaching supervision. The chapter provides an overview of the various definitions of coaching supervision from selected literature and accreditation agencies. The often perplexing issues of how things are similar and different are explored. Coaching, mentoring, ICF mentor coaching and coaching supervision are differentiated. The chapter describes the functions of coaching supervision as they are seen in the literature and as we would describe them in Solution Focused coaching supervision. Core standards and competencies of coaching supervision as they have been developed by the respective credentialing agencies are presented in a synopsis and you can learn how Solution Focused coaching supervision aligns with them, as well as how it goes beyond.

Chapter 3 delves into the foundations, epistemology, axiology and theory of change of Solution Focused practice as it pertains to Solution Focused coaching supervision. Its roots in social constructionist, post-structuralist and postmodern thoughts are delineated. How Solution Focused coaching supervision demonstrates adherence to these systems of thought is presented through the "Galveston Declaration", a declaration of Solution Focused, narrative and collaborative practitioners on the preferences of their practice contrasted with more traditional psychological approaches. While this is a chapter that may seem high on academia and philosophy (which we admit it is), it is also grounded in and relevant to the everyday practice of coaching supervision. The Solution Focused approach was developed by respecting and learning about what ordinary people with aspirations find beneficial to live their ordinary extraordinary lives. This tradition has continued into Solution Focused coaching supervision: what do so-called ordinary coaches need from coaching supervision so that they can live their brilliance and make their significant contribution to creating landscapes in which their coaching supervision clients can be at their best, providing hope and progress filled coaching?

In Chapter 4, the reader learns about the coaching supervision "moves" a Solution Focused coaching supervisor can use during a supervision session. The Solution Focused coaching supervisor prefers to use interactional metaphors such as dance moves, rather than technicist metaphors such as "tools" and "techniques". The metaphor of the "Art Gallery Walk" which provides a possible useful structure for a coaching supervision session is explored. Other moves of the coaching supervisor and the coaching supervision client are described as per the functions of the coaching supervision. Some concrete examples are provided for how Solution Focused coaching supervisors might respond when called to provide assistance in one of the coaching supervision functions.

Chapter 5 breathes life into how coaching supervision can support coaches to demonstrate ethical coaching practice. It offers the Solution Focused resource activation stance to exploring ethical dilemmas, encouraging data-based decision-making, while not losing sight of the fact that people are in conversation and in relationships. Responding to ethical dilemmas is framed as an opportunity for coaching supervision clients to become clearer about standards of practice, about how to respond to complexity, ambiguity and uncertainty with creativity and ingenuity that is grounded in what the coaching supervision client wants to be known for, and the quality and integrity of their communication with their coaching clients. A pragmatic approach, anchored in the awareness of the coaching Codes of Ethics, and tempered by rigour and compassion is offered as a way to resolve ethical dilemmas with a Solution Focused perspective.

Chapter 6 has a more specific focus than individual coaching supervision in that it focuses on the exploration of specific client cases, to enhance the quality of service to a particular client. This chapter describes how the Solution Focused tenets of pragmatism, curiosity, taking an interactional view and seeing progress and resources rather than deficits apply when offering case supervision. The differences between ICF mentor coaching and coaching supervision when reviewing a recording of a coaching session are described. The chapter offers an annotated transcript of a Solution Focused case supervision session to illustrate these ideas with a coaching supervision client who is stuck and wants advice from the coaching supervisor.

Chapter 7 dives into how to respond as a coaching supervisor when requested to supervise a coaching supervision client who draws on a different coaching model/approach from the coaching supervisor. Solution Focused coaching supervision, with its emphasis on client goals and strengths and restraint when it comes to interpretations and advice, is especially suited to collaborating with supervision clients from different approaches. This chapter offers some practical tips as well as a transcript of a session between a Solution Focused coaching supervisor and a coaching supervision client whose coaching is embedded in Transactional Analysis.

Chapter 8 alerts readers to the fact that there is no generalisable development of coach maturity in foreseeable stages and that growth as a coach can be recognised by different signals. The chapter makes use of the findings of Scott Miller et al. (2020) on raising the effectiveness of psychotherapy by "deliberate practice" and allows coaching supervisors to utilise similar techniques for the growth and development of coaching supervision clients. Deliberate practice allows coaching supervisors to support coaching supervision clients to discover and grow towards their individual learning goals as supported by their coaching clients' feedback through an adapted Outcome Rating Scale (Miller & Duncan, 2000) and the Session Rating Scale (Miller, Duncan & Johnson, 2002).

Chapter 9 provides a short overview of the history of reflective practice. The chapter also contains a summary of the most prevalent models of reflective practice. The chapter also provides guidance on how to embed reflection in the coaching supervision process.

Chapter 10 is devoted to ICF mentor coaching because mentoring and mentor coaching are located as overlapping with coaching supervision in purpose and function. Mentoring describes the relationship between a person with more expertise and experience who supports the aspirations of someone in their career development. Mention is made of the EMCC's stance on mentoring. ICF mentor coaching is located as a subset of coaching supervision. It has a very specific purpose and set of requirements that must be complied with. ICF mentor coaching forms part of the ICF gold standard quality framework. The role, competencies, duties and responsibilities are outlined. It focuses on the ongoing development of a coach's ability to demonstrate the ICF core competencies in their coaching. The chapter foregrounds a vital function of coaching supervision and ICF mentor coaching, namely, the generating and giving of feedback – both written and verbal. Attention is paid to the complex task that ICF mentor coaches face in providing feedback that is both quality assurance informed, as well as focused on the development of coaching capability. This includes the management of bias and/or blindspots. Extracts from a transcript are offered to illustrate ICF mentor coaching in action.

Coaching supervision groups are often seen as a cost-effective way to provide coaching supervision. However, this is only one of the many benefits of group coaching supervision as compared with individual coaching supervision. Chapter 11 outlines the benefits as well as the challenges of coaching supervision groups and offers ideas for how to manage them. The contracting process for how to set up a group is described, covering the aspects that are similar to setting up an individual coaching supervision contract, as well as specific issues that need to be attended to in a group. Examples of Solution Focused questions are given to support the coaching supervisor enable the group to explore their best hopes for and from the group, as well as enabling the group to co-create roles within the group and take responsibility for their learning. The Solution Focused coaching supervision moves outlined earlier in the book are adapted to the context of coaching supervision groups. The Solution Focused reflecting team format for presenting cases in a group is outlined and includes a transcript of a group coaching supervision session using this process to bring this to life. Many new coaching supervisors may feel nervous about supervising groups, so the chapter contains reflective exercises to help build the skills needed as a group coaching supervisor.

Chapter 12 deals with "Peer Coaching Supervision". The terms "peer coaching supervision" and "intervision" are both used to describe a peer-led group engaged by coaches who each contribute knowledge, skills and experience and support each other to learn and grow from one another's coaching practice. There is no designated leader, rather a sense of equity, commitment to generating benefit for all, and self-organisation are characteristic of the fabric of these groups. This chapter starts by outlining the differences inherent in these names – "supervision" implying vision from above, compared with "intervision" meaning between, among, reciprocally or together. Peer supervision can occur in reciprocal pairs or a peer supervision chain process as well as in a group format. The benefits and challenges of this form of coaching supervision are discussed, using examples of Solution Focused questions to help maximise the benefits and minimise the challenges. The process of co-creating a well-functioning peer coaching supervision process is outlined including establishing the "why" or purpose of the group, followed by the what, when, where and how. Examples of peer coaching supervision groups in action are shared.

"Coaching Supervision for Team Coaches" (Chapter 13) starts by defining team coaching and its supervision, emphasising the unique aspects of the Solution Focused approach. Unlike traditional approaches, the focus will be on the coaching supervision client rather than their team coaching clients, steering clear of external analyses and diagnoses. The chapter navigates through the differences between individual coaching supervision and team coaching supervision, as well as the distinctions from group coaching supervision. It presents compelling reasons for engaging in team coaching supervision and outlines potential strategies for effective coaching supervision. Challenges inherent in team coaching supervision are explored, including considerations for supervisors dealing with diverse coaching methods, the delicate balance between guiding and advising, and the introspective aspect of self within the coaching supervision process. It also offers some strategies to supervise a team and the team coach together. The chapter aims to provide aspiring as well as experienced coaching supervisors with insights and tools for navigating the nuanced landscape of Solution Focused team coaching supervision.

The next chapter is "Common Topics Arising in Coaching Supervision". While each coaching supervision client brings topics and concerns that are unique, there are many common topics and challenges that a coaching supervisor may need to deal with. This chapter lists some of these, including a coaching supervision client feeling stuck and always wanting advice, a coaching supervision client not seeing the value of coaching supervision; a coaching supervision client constantly feeling inadequate; a coaching supervision client showing negative bias towards their coaching clients; a coaching supervision client focusing only on their coaching clients and not their own professional growth. This chapter brings together all the learning across the book, to help the coaching supervisor to use Solution Focused questions and moves to deal with these topics. As well as drawing on transcripts from earlier in the book where some of these topics are illustrated, additional examples are shared. The coaching supervisor is invited to apply these ideas to their own work via questions and activities for reflection and action.

The last chapter "Suppose a Miracle Happened – Our Preferred Future for Coaching Supervision" offers an outlook into the future of Solution Focused and social constructionist coaching supervision. What we call "on the horizon" or "going beyond" topics, as well as opportunities for future research and possibilities to further develop the practice of coaching supervision, are discussed.

How to Read This Book

You do not necessarily have to read this book from the front to the back cover – feel free to browse around and read what is interesting or useful to you at the time. We would recommend that you read the introduction to coaching supervision and the introduction to Solution Focused supervision first as these chapters introduce some foundational ideas without which it will be difficult to gain full benefit from the subsequent chapters.

This book was written to be a companion for coaching supervisors committed to expanding the quality of their own coaching supervision, as well providing a significantly value-adding experience for their coaching supervision clients. While this book respects and supports the compliance aspects of coaching supervision adopted by the accreditation agencies, it aspires to inspire coaching supervisors and their coaching supervision clients to go beyond compliance to enjoyment, fulfilment and ongoing learning and growth.

References

Miller, S.D., & Duncan, B.L. (2000). *The Outcome Rating Scale*. Author.

Miller, S.D., Duncan, B.L. & Johnson, L.D. (2002). *The Session Rating Scale 3.0*. Author.

Miller, S.D., Hubble, M.A. & Chow, D. (2020). *Better Results: Using Deliberate Practice to Improve Therapeutic Effectiveness*. American Psychological Association. https://doi.org/10.1037/0000191-000

2 Introduction to Coaching Supervision

Kirsten Dierolf and Svea van der Hoorn

Introduction

This chapter provides an overview of the field of coaching supervision to date. It offers a short history of supervision and describes several strands of its origin as well as a history of the recent developments towards coaching supervision, together with various definitions of coaching supervision from selected literature and accreditation agencies. Coaching, mentoring, International Coaching Federation (ICF) mentor coaching and coaching supervision are differentiated. The chapter describes the functions of coaching supervision as they are seen in the literature and as we would describe them in Solution Focused coaching supervision. Core standards and competencies of coaching supervision as they have been developed by the respective credentialing agencies are presented in a synopsis, and the reader can learn how Solution Focused coaching supervision aligns with them.

A Brief Look at the History of Supervision

"Supervision" can be considered a family resemblance term: many fields use the term, and the meaning can vary from "control" to "partnership" and anything in between, and something else still. Before we look at definitions of coaching supervision, we would therefore like to have a brief look at the multiple strands of history that are relevant for coaching supervision.

In most fields, "supervision" started as an effort to control performance or finances. In the United States of America, "supervision" was used in the education system to ensure quality of instruction in the early 1800s. In the precursors of social work in Europe, "supervision" was used to control money spent by welfare agents such as volunteer organisations. Clinical supervision in psychotherapy started as a teaching and quality insurance endeavour for psychoanalysts which included a personal teaching analysis for the students. With the advent of industrialisation, "supervision" also came to mean performance control within organisations (Belardi, 1994).

Starting in the 1950s the focus of supervision shifted. In Germany, reflections on the horrors of the holocaust and the command-and-control system and mindset that made it possible led the social sciences to move towards

DOI: 10.4324/9781003390527-2

collaboration and consultation in supervision. In the United Kingdom, a form of peer supervision started in 1950 known as Balint groups, founded by Michael Balint. The focus of these groups was to encourage physicians to explore themselves and generate insights in a psychoanalytic group process so as to offer relationship-centred care (Balint, 1985). Other group supervision formats appeared with the humanistic philosophy's influence on psychotherapy. These group supervision formats were less about understanding subconscious mechanisms but more about support for the medical practitioners and encouraging partnership between the medical practitioner and client. Expert knowledge was stressed less. In Germany, supervision entered the organisational world around 1980, as a form of support and development for people working in and with organisations: consultants, leaders, coaches (if they used that term then). The German association for supervision (which changed its name to German association for supervision and coaching recently) was founded in 1989 (DGSv, 2024).

"Coaching Supervision" is a relatively new practice which has developed significantly over the last years and has established itself as a discipline separate from coaching. A definition of coaching supervision as a profession containing scope, purpose and functions, practices and more would normally be the task of academics and peer-reviewed journals (Bachkirova et al., 2020, p. 31). In the case of coaching supervision, practitioner literature and coaching associations were faster in placing definitions into the public domain. One perhaps unhelpful by-product of this is that definitions of coaching supervision lacked attention to their philosophical, epistemological and change theory homes. This has created a dilemma for comparisons of definitions, and the appropriateness of their application to all and any coaching practice, each of which will have its own philosophical, epistemological and change theory home. Discordance arises when comparisons are made between coaching supervision approaches embedded in, for example, positivist psychology, adult learning, pragmatics of communication and social constructionism. In the following, we would like to share a few of the definitions from academic and practitioner literature, as well as from coaching associations.

Definitions of Coaching Supervision

Some Definitions From Literature

The following list is by no means intended to be complete or even current as the field is developing rapidly and new definitions emerge almost every few months. We have selected the below to show a range. Note that not all authors use the specifier "coaching" but rather the more general "supervision". We will illuminate Solution Focused coaching supervision in relation to each definition.

> Supervision can (…) provide a key process to help a living profession or organization breathe and learn.
>
> (Hawkins & Shohet, 2012, p. 237)

The Solution Focused approach also sees coaching supervision mainly as a process which can help an organisation learn. Supervision is a way in which the supervision client and the organisation can develop. If a coaching supervisor is working with more than one coach in an organisation, their feedback on commonly experienced topics can be very valuable to the organisations. Such feedback honours confidentiality agreements with individual and team clients by offering themes in the language of the organisations' vision, mission and targets, rather than being linked to specific content expressed in coaching sessions.

> Supervision is a forum where supervisees review and reflect on their work in order to do it better
>
> (Carroll, 2007, p. 433)

> Coaching supervision provides "a working alliance between two professionals where coaches offer an account of their work, reflect on it, receive feedback and receive guidance – if appropriate".
>
> (Inskipp & Proctor, 1993, p. 28)

The focus in these definitions is on the alliance or working relationship and the work of the supervision client who "offers an account, reviews and reflects". This is very close to the Solution Focused understanding of coaching supervision as a partnership between a more experienced and a less experienced coach. The supervision client does most of the work, the supervisor gives feedback and provides guidance only if appropriate. In Solution Focused coaching supervision, the appropriateness would hinge most strongly on whether feedback or guidance are asked for by the coaching supervision client, or there was a clear alert about ethical conduct and/or accurate interpretation and implementation of a coaching approach in what the coaching supervision client is describing.

> Supervision is the process by which a coach/mentor/consultant, with the help of the supervisor, who is not working directly with the client, can attend to understanding better both the client system and themselves as part of the client-coach/mentor system, and transform their work.
>
> (Hawkins & Smith, 2006, p. 147)

Here, the coaching supervisor's role is seen as someone with an outside perspective who can help the supervision client to "better understand the client system and themselves". The focus is on understanding as if from the outside. While a coaching supervisor will have different experiences from the coaching supervision client and may be able to offer perspectives which are less influenced by a direct interaction with the coaching client, these perspectives would not be offered as a way to "understand the client" in Solution

Focused coaching supervision. As mentioned in our chapter on theory, Solution Focused coaching supervision would not in any way analyse the coaching client or aim to "understand" them. The interactions between coaching supervisor and the coaching supervision client are the relevant unit or system for coaching supervision.

> Coaching supervision is a formal process of professional support, which ensures continuing development of the coach and effectiveness of his/ her coaching practice through interactive reflection, interpretative evaluation and the sharing of expertise.
>
> (Bachkirova, 2008, pp. 16–17)

This definition also integrates the objective of coaching supervision: the continuous development of the coach and effectiveness of their coaching practice. This fits very well with Solution Focused thinking which sees coaching supervision as an outcomes-oriented activity. How we notice that coaching supervision is working is when the coach develops into the coach they want to be, when their coaching aligns with coaching standards and when their practice is effective for their clients. While reflection and sharing of expertise would be part of a Solution Focused definition of coaching supervision practice, "interpretive evaluation" is probably less so, depending on what that practice looks like. The Solution Focused approach is less focused on explanations and evaluation and more focused on progress and collaboration (see Chapter 3).

Definitions by Coaching Accreditation Agencies

All of the major coaching accreditation agencies have published their own definitions of coaching supervision. Some also have produced coaching supervision competency frameworks which we will cover later in this chapter. We start by providing you with definitions and our reflections on how the definitions offered by coaching accreditation agencies fit with a social constructionist, Solution Focused view of coaching supervision.

European Mentoring and Coaching Council (EMCC)

> The term "supervision" describes the process by which the work and well-being of the coach/mentor is overseen and advice/guidance sought. Supervision with a properly trained supervisor provides space and time to reflect on professional functioning in complex situations. Supervisors focus on the ongoing personal development of coaches/ mentors to enable them to deliver best practice with their clients.
>
> (EMCC, 2015, p. 2)

The focus is on the well-being of the coach, reflection and personal development to deliver quality benchmarked practice in complex situations.

The verb that is being used here is "overseen". In a Solution Focused coaching supervision definition, we would stress the partnership between the coaching supervisor and the coaching supervision client in determining the quality assurance aspect of the coaching supervision practice.

Association for Coaching (AC)

> Coaching supervision is a formal and protected time for facilitating in depth reflection for coaches to discuss their work with someone who is experienced as a coach. Supervision offers a confidential framework within a collaborative working relationship in which the practice, tasks, process and challenges of the coaching work can be explored. (Accredited Coaching Supervisor Applicant Guide.
>
> The primary functions of supervision are to support, develop and ensure ethical and quality benchmarked practice of coaches in service of their coaching clients (individuals and organisations) and their professional associations. Supervision is not a "policing" role, but rather a "trusting and collegial professional relationship".
>
> (Association for Coaching, 2018, p. 3)

The AC's definition focuses on partnership and collaboration and integrates all but one of the functions of supervision that we would also stress in Solution Focused coaching supervision: exploration of practice, process, tasks, challenges, supporting the coach and their ethically informed practice. Solution Focused coaching supervision would add strengths of the coach.

Association for Professional Executive Coaching & Supervision (APECS)

> Each Executive Coach will choose a form of supervision and a supervisor that best fits their learning needs. In ongoing and regular supervision they will discuss confidentially their thoughts, feelings and reactions to their work at all levels: clients, relationships, interventions, contracts, impasses, joys, upsets etc. Supervision will be a forum for reflection on coaching work where supervisees will take responsibility for their own learning. Supervisors will provide APECS with a short annual report on supervisees assuring APECS that they are working ethically and to an acceptable standard.
>
> (APECS, n.d.)

APECS stresses that supervision clients take responsibility for their own learning which we also support as Solution Focused coaching supervisors. The word "joys" in the description of what will be discussed in coaching supervision is close to the Solution Focused inclusion of reflecting on strengths and things that are already going well. In Solution Focused supervision one major topic will be what the supervision client already is doing well and what brings them joy and contentment in their work.

Association of Coaching Supervisors (AOCS)

> Supervision on a 1–1 or group basis is the formal opportunity for coaches working with clients to share, in confidence, their caseload activity to gain insight, support and direction for themselves and thereby enabling them to better work in the service of their clients
>
> (Association of Coaching Supervisors, n.d.)

AOCS has a definition of minimal elegance and a focus on self-directedness, which Solution Focused coaching supervision shares. Solution Focused coaching supervision draws on the concept of Occam's Razor – keep things simple and grounded by shaving away as many assumptions as possible. We note the word "case load" which seems to assume something heavy. In our experience both the "load" and the "lightness" of the supervision client's practice are topics appropriate for reflection in coaching supervision.

International Coaching Federation (ICF)

> Coaching Supervision is a collaborative learning practice to continually build the capacity of the coach through reflective dialogue for the benefit of both coaches and clients. Coaching Supervision focuses on the development of the coach's capacity through offering a richer and broader opportunity for support and development. Coaching Supervision creates a safe environment for the coach to share their successes and failures in becoming masterful in the way they work with their clients.
>
> (ICF, n.d.)

The ICF definition of coaching supervision is aligned with Solution Focused coaching supervision as focusing on sharing "successes", being "a collaborative learning practice" and with the aim of "building the capacity of the coach … for the benefit of both coaches and clients". Where the ICF definition speaks of "offering a richer and broader opportunity for support and development", Solution Focused coaching supervision more specifically refers to "resource detecting" for "change talk" and "possibility talk". The ICF is a fairly late adopter of coaching supervision as desirable or necessary to establishing and maintaining quality in coaching. Mentor coaching has been a focus for the ICF (ICF, n.d.)

At this time (2024), the ICF requires 10 hours of mentor coaching as opposed to coaching supervision for all individual coaching credential applications. Coaching supervision is required by ICF only for the Advanced Certificate in Team Coaching (ACTC). However, ICF is also moving towards recognising coaching supervision as an important part of coach development and a competency framework and certification are work in progress.

Supervision, Coaching, Mentor Coaching, Mentoring – What Is What?

Another way of defining coaching supervision can be through its differentiation from other modalities like coaching, mentor coaching or mentoring. A quip heard from Svea van der Hoorn goes like this: Question: "Why must there be a gherkin in every bowl of olives?" Answer: "So that the olives can know that they are olives". Often, we know things by distinction – what they are not – more easily than by what they are. In the following we would like to provide our view on the differentiating factors between the above-mentioned modalities. Of course, what is being communicated when someone uses these words always depends on how they are using the word and the context. So, if a potential client is asking for "mentor coaching", they might well mean "coaching supervision" and vice versa. A good contracting conversation will include exploring what support and development service the client is looking for by enquiring about purpose, process and outcome expectations.

Coaching

Participants in our supervision coaching training courses are sometimes quite surprised that the Solution Focused coaching supervision process is not much different from a coaching process. Indeed, the structure, questions, comments, the way the practitioner partners with the supervision client may well be experienced as more similar than different. What makes coaching supervision different from coaching is the range of topics that the supervision client may bring and their expectations of the purpose, process and outcomes. Coaching supervision is limited to coaches as clients, and the topics of coaching supervision are the development and well-being of the coach, in relation to their coaching practice and ability to serve their clients rather than in relation to other aspects, for example, their parenting skills, ability to find a romantic partner, their ability to decide upon how to engage with social media. The latter is an example of a grey area topic that some coaching supervisors will engage with as part of providing support for the business development of the coach's coaching practice. Another differentiating factor is that a coaching supervisor who does have knowledge and experience in relation to their coaching supervision client's topic may offer this if desired by the coaching supervision client. The quality assurance aspect is also stronger in coaching supervision than it is in coaching. Is there a sharp line between coaching and coaching supervision, with more difference than similarity? Solution Focused coaching supervisors will likely think "no".

Mentoring

Mentoring as it is understood in many EMCC circles relates to coaching supervision in similar ways as coaching mentioned above (see, for example, Clutterbuck, 2022 or Garvey & Stokes, 2021). Mentoring is seen as a sibling to coaching and closer to coaching supervision in that a mentor will offer their own perspective to the mentoring/supervision client rather than relying mainly on questions and observations. ICF circles differentiate "coaching" and "mentoring", sometimes almost with an air of superiority of "pure coaching" which needs to be demonstrated in the ICF performance evaluations for a credential. If the word "mentoring" is used by a client, a coach or coach supervisor is well advised to ask what kind of support the client wants: the use of the word is very muddled and even politicised unhelpfully.

Mentor Coaching

ICF offers this definition:

> Mentor Coaching for an ICF Credential consists of coaching and feedback in a collaborative, appreciative and dialogued process based on an observed or recorded coaching session to increase the coach's capability in coaching, in alignment with the ICF Core Competencies.
>
> (ICF Mentor Coaching, n.d.)

In some communities, "mentor coaching" is used synonymously with coaching supervision. It is understood as being about a coach being "mentored" by a more experienced coach, who is already at or beyond the credential level being applied for. The ICF has created a special usage of the phrase. An ICF "mentor coach" discusses a coaching recording with a coach in light of the coach's desire to obtain an ICF credential. In the mentor coaching session, coach and mentor talk about how the recording demonstrates the ICF coaching core competencies at the credential level that the coach is aspiring to (Associate Certified Coach, Professional Certified Coach or Master Certified Coach). The mentor coach both offers feedback and coaches. We suggest using "ICF mentor coaching" when referring to this type of mentoring.

EMCC is ambivalent when it comes to whether to recognise ICF mentor coaching as "coaching supervision" or not. In our opinion, ICF mentor coaching could be seen as a sub-category of coaching supervision. In coaching supervision, the supervisor and coaching supervision client may discuss a coaching recording in reference to a competency framework, if the coaching supervision client desires this, and if it seems useful for their development in relation to standards of coaching practice.

Functions of Supervision

We have touched upon the topic of the functions of supervision as part of the definition of coaching supervision. As there are many definitions of coaching supervision, there are also many different understandings of the functions of supervision. We have listed a few below (a selection, by no means an extensive and encompassing list):

Proctor (1986)

- Normative
- Formative
- Restorative

Kadushin (1976)

- Managerial
- Educational
- Supportive

Hawkins and Smith (2006)

- Qualitative
- Developmental
- Resourcing

Lucas and Larcombe (2016)

- Ethical
- Technical
- Personal
- Commercial

The functions of supervision tend to fall into a few categories. One function that is consistently mentioned is the supportive function which focuses on the well-being of the coaching supervision client. In coaching supervision, the coaching supervision client can receive support in any aspect of their work, which may be experienced as emotionally difficult, straining or otherwise impacting their well-being.

The ethical dimension of the coaching supervision client's practice is also a topic in coaching supervision and the function of the coaching supervision is to guide the coaching supervision client towards engaging in ethical coaching practice. The coaching supervision client can reflect on any ethical issues they may be concerned about and explore them and receive guidance from the coaching supervisor.

Coaching supervision also serves as a quality insurance. Coaching supervision clients talk about what is going well and not so well in their practice and, by engaging with a coaching supervisor, they are supported in their learning journey to become better coaches. We would not see the quality insurance aspect of coaching supervision as a directive or punitive interaction. By engaging in coaching supervision the coaching supervision client will grow in their competence and hence confidence, which will automatically result in the coaching supervision client's growth in quality.

Another function of coaching supervision is supporting the personal growth of the coaching supervision client which happens when someone reflects on their work and how it affects them and their clients.

The last function managerial and commercial are seldom mentioned as functions of coaching supervision. However, building your business as a coach and being a coaching entrepreneur can affect both the coaching supervision' client's well-being and their performance. Hence these topics can be the focus of coaching supervision. In our view, if a coaching supervision focuses only on business development aspects, it would probably fall more neatly into the modality of consulting, mentoring or coaching (depending on the amount of advice given).

Core Standards and Competencies of Coach Supervision

Development and Philosophies of Competence Frameworks

EMCC and ICF have similar but somewhat different approaches to the generation of standards or core competencies for their respective accreditations. In the following we describe what we know from what is available in the public domain and in the ICF and EMCC communities.

ICF

ICF follows a job analysis process conducted by a company specialised in generating core competencies for organisations. Job analysis is generally used in organisations when it comes to the description of core tasks of a function. Learning and development activities are built on the identified capabilities, and performance management and succession planning is carried out by measuring people's performance against the generated competencies. The ICF has used this method previously for generating updated coaching core competencies.

The ICF core competencies for coaching supervision were defined using this process. A team of experienced coaching supervisors generated a definition of coaching supervision. The work group at the level of ICF Global designed a survey with multiple statements around supervision knowledge, skills and abilities. The survey was distributed to all ICF members and beyond. Everyone was encouraged to contribute and share perspectives. Based on the data collected a clustering of information was performed. That clustering was brought to the first session of a specialised work group formed by Subject Matter Experts (SMEs), who were gathered across organisations, continents and cultures and coaching models/approaches. The SMEs were invited to reflect upon the listing in relation to what happens in coaching supervision in order to distinguish coaching supervision from mentor coaching. This provided the opportunity to observe and extract the skills, knowledge and abilities that are most important to coaching supervisors. Through multiple workshops, a set of coaching supervision core competencies was refined and restructured.

This draft set is to be evaluated by the ICF Board. As at 2024, the SMEs agreed that there is still work to be done to further refine the coaching supervision core competencies.

EMCC

EMCC followed a similar working group approach, but with a group of academics developing a set of core standards. This was then discussed with the wider community and refined. The EMCC supervision framework is not restricted to being coach specific, rather it is designed to be relevant to supervision for mentors and coaches. With this in mind, we will use the term "supervision" rather than "coaching supervision" in reference to the EMCC framework. EMCC writes:

> A Note on Competence Frameworks
>
> EMCC supports the use of competence frameworks as part of a broader approach to the training, development and assessment of coaches, mentors and supervisors. The EMCC Supervision Competence Framework describes the skills and behaviours we believe to be associated with good practice in supervision. EMCC also recognises that competence frameworks have limitations and that there are some qualities of an effective supervisor that are difficult to define. Supervision is, essentially, a relational process. Please bear this in mind when working with this document.
>
> The capability indicators listed below each competence are for guidance only. They are intended to stimulate dialogue and enable reflection; they are not a checklist of specific requirements for effective supervision.
>
> (EMCC, 2019, p. 8)

The EMCC's description of supervision as a relational process seems much more in line with social constructionist approaches than the ICF process which aims at the description of almost reified competencies which a good supervisor needs to have. In social constructionist philosophy, "a competence" or "a skill" would not be described as a thing that the practitioner has. If we use the words: "This supervisor has this competence", we would be speaking about our prediction of what they might be able to do in the future based on our past observation of the person.

A Synopsis of Competence Frameworks

In the following you will find a synopsis of the competence frameworks as they are at the time of the publication of this book. As these competency frameworks may be changing during the time of the publication of this book, we want to present a synopsis rather than presenting the overlapping competencies and standards of the various accreditation agencies. We are describing the competencies and standards as well as how Solution Focused supervision demonstrates these competencies.

Builds and Maintains Relationship

Solution Focus concurs that coaching supervision is a relational activity. A supervision session is a conversation between an experienced practitioner and a supervision client who would like to reflect on their work with the aim of personal and professional growth. Solution Focused supervision, just like any other form of Solution Focused or social construction practice, focuses on how together they can co-create something that is meaningful and useful for the supervision client. The focus is on value creation, with the relationship being almost a by-product, rather than something that the supervisor needs to work at establishing. Whereas many supervision approaches consider the relationship to be a site of potential tension and even conflict, in Solution Focused supervision there is no idea of possible resistance by the client to ideas, interpretations or observations from the supervisor. The Solution Focused supervisor does not entertain hypotheses or otherwise analyse the client. Generally, Solution Focused supervisors are interested in what their supervision clients want and what they already know about possibilities and resources that can move them there. This focus on strengths and desired outcomes/best hopes creates an appreciative atmosphere in the supervision which in turn sustains the trust and safety that the parties bring by contracting to engage in supervision together. Resistance is seen as an opportunity for the supervisor to learn more about what the supervision client desires and their ideas about how to move towards their best hopes (De Shazer, 1984).

With the focus on hopes and desired outcomes, the Solution Focused supervisor is also highly attuned to what contribution the supervision client would like the supervisor to make to the supervision. If the supervision client would like to talk about an emotionally straining event, the supervisor will support. If the client would like to develop a skill, the supervisor will coach or even teach. The relationship will always be one of regarding the client as resourceful and capable of developing the improvements they desire.

Supports the Well-Being of the Supervision Client

Solution Focused supervision by definition creates a supportive space for the supervision client. In any form of social constructionist practice, the supervisor is asked to provide a space where they are de-centred, but influential. We recognise the paradox in this and see it as enabling creativity, learning and growth. The supervision client is in the centre, yet the supervisor is fully present as a human being, which fosters an atmosphere of openness. Different social constructionist practices vary in their degree of practitioners' self-disclosure during the practice. Solution Focused practice favours a strong centring of the client. Narrative practice also works with practitioners' resonances to what the supervision client is experiencing. Collaborative practices focus very strongly on the collaboration of both practitioner and client with little restraint on the practitioners' self-disclosure. In all cases, an atmosphere of acceptance and openness is co-created.

Accreditation agencies' competences and standard models also mention psychological safety as important. As Solution Focused practice is not about "the inside" or "the psyche" of the client which needs to "feel safe" but about the interactions, we would translate "psychological safety" into "interactional safety". As described above, Solution Focused supervision provides a safe space via the supervisor's stance of radical acceptance and acting from an interactional perspective when so-called resistance is experienced by either or both parties.

Manages the Contract

The supervision competencies and standards of the accrediting agencies mention the importance of a flexible contracting process encompassing all stakeholders – the "supervision client system". In Solution Focused supervision perspective change questions like: "Suppose our supervision process is successful, what will your relevant stakeholders notice that is better?" take care of integrating the various perspectives into the supervision process. Depending on the situation, a supervisor may also speak to the organisation they are providing supervision for and integrate their perspectives into the supervision.

There are some cases of mandated supervision clients, for example when supervision is the requirement from one of the accreditation agencies for the retention of a coaching credential. In these cases the Solution Focused supervisor will invite the supervision client to work on the topics that allow the supervision client to retain the credential by asking questions like: "what would this accreditation agency need to see you do or be so that they would be comfortable to grant/renew/reinstate your credential?" The supervisor will always invite the supervision client to work on what the supervision client wants to work on and never impose any topic on the client. Solution Focused supervision is always voluntary, even if it is mandated. While the client may be mandated to take supervision, the topics that are discussed should be topics that that supervision client is interested and working on.

Duty of Care in the Contract

Duty of care is a term that is more familiar to practitioners who have statutory or safe-guarding responsibilities. However, in most civil societies, care for a stranger in need is seen as an act of compassion, not an interference or restriction of the person's rights and freedoms. In supervision, duty of care is related to supporting the well-being of both the supervision client and their clients. This can be done through reflection and decision-making on a variety of topics, such as scope and remit of practice, appropriateness of qualifications and training to undertake particular work, ethical concerns and dilemmas, as well as reminders and guidance about taking into consideration standards of practice, local laws, customs and norms, and organisational policies and procedures. In this way supervision acts as a safety net where the supervision client can engage with duty of care in ways that promote learning and growth rather than in an atmosphere of blame and correction. Solution Focused supervisors often enquire "you must have good reasons for what you are doing/ what you decided .... what are your good reasons?" The Solution Focused supervisor will then engage in a conversation which begins with seeing the supervision client as competent and resourceful and then moving into talk about "what instead" possibilities. Thus, perspective is expanded to allow for more complex consideration about the factors the supervision client needs to respond to.

Promotes and Executes Ethical Behaviour

Coaching supervision also has a quality assurance function. In the fulfilment of this function the coaching supervisor may notice that their supervision client acts in ways that conflict with the ethical standards of the accreditation agencies and/or generally accepted ethical practice when involved in people development. In this case, the competencies and standards of the accreditation agencies require the coaching supervisor to act as an ethical sounding board and to invite awareness of the ethical codes of conduct on the part of the coaching supervision client.

The coaching supervisor needs to know about ethical frameworks and also needs to model ethical behaviour in their own practice. The above described way of aligning coaching supervision clients' goals with mandated goals for supervision also work very well here. The Solution Focused supervisor will mention the code of ethics and inquire about the supervision clients' response rather than shaming or blaming the client, thereby modelling ethical behaviour themselves.

Coaching supervisors do not have the luxury of confidentiality mandated by law in most jurisdictions. They can be called to testify about supervision sessions in front of courts of law. It is very important that coaching supervision clients know about this limitation on confidentiality and also know about the duty of care of the supervisor. As part of contracting it promotes sound ethical practice of the coaching supervisor proactively enquires about any statutory requirements, policy directives or local laws, customs and norms that should be taken into consideration during the coaching supervision. In particular attention needs to be paid to information sharing with stakeholders other than the person the supervision client is coaching. Coaching supervisors are encouraged to put in place expanded confidentiality agreements, rather than narrow confidentiality agreements. For example, rather than start a coaching session with openers like "I want to assure our sessions are confidential, what is said here stays here", coaching supervisors can encourage more explicit and transparent confidentiality arrangements. For example,

> I want to assure you that I wish to respect your privacy and to do that I'd like to discuss with you that you are free to discuss what you say in these sessions with anyone else that you think can support you in the learning and growth that brings you to coaching. I, however, will not be discussing what we say without requesting your permission. I would like you to know that there might be circumstances under which my duty of care obligation would make it appropriate for me to share information without your in the moment permission. This usually happens when I become concerned for your well being or the well being of others. An example could be if you were taken ill during a session and I was concerned that you might require medical attention. Let's discuss whether you are willing to enter into coaching with an expanded confidentiality agreement?

It is common then to engage in a discussion with the coaching supervision client about how they go about establishing with their coaching clients what the terms and conditions are for sharing information, for storage of information and for whom to contact in case of an emergency or concern about safety and well-being. In Solution Focused coaching supervision this is linked to supporting the client to reflect on who is already part of their learning and growth journey, and who else might they want to include, whether as supports to prevent things from getting worse, as people who can assist them to cope with current circumstances, and as people who can be part of noticing and celebrating progress.

Self-awareness

"Self"-awareness is somewhat of a strange concept for social constructionist approaches. There may be an idea of a self-reflecting on the self. An emotion, for example, in social-constructionist terms, would not be something internal that a person could analyse like an internal object. Rather, a sentence like: "I am angry" would be seen as opening a language trap in comparison to "He is angry" or "I am in my living room". In order to determine whether a sentence like "He is angry" or "I am in my living room" is true, we would need criteria. The angry person is red in the face and shouting. The room that I am in has a table and a sofa, and is generally used for relaxing. These kinds of criteria do not exist when we are talking about our own emotions. When I say: "I am angry", I am not describing my emotion but I am avowing it. As a child I learned to replace my expression of anger, for example throwing myself on the floor and pounding it with my little fists, by saying: "I am angry", which is undoubtedly more pleasant for the people around me. This in turn is probably why I was taught to replace the tantrum with words.

"Self"-awareness, in social constructionist terms, does not have anything to do with the analysis and processing of one's internal processes. In order to make use of the term, we might look at situations in which it is used. When other approaches talk about self-awareness of the supervisor, several sub-competencies or standards are mentioned that we can make sense of because they have a home in lived experience.

The ICF speaks of awareness of one's own biases. Part of self-awareness seems to be the ability to distinguish what pertains to the situation at hand and what may be influences of our past that cloud our experience of the present moment. This fits quite well with a social constructionist lens. We are shaped by our experiences, by our interactions with people and our environment. We tell ourselves stories based on our past and our expectations of the future are shaped in part by our past. In social construction self-awareness may be rooted in the openness for alternative stories and the acceptance of the present moment. It is quite ironic that the ability to accept what is, to be non-judgemental and open for different outcomes and interpretations which is built into social constructionist approaches as an everyday and ordinary human capability, is deemed an outcome of years of self-reflection, encounter groups, supervisory therapy and more in other approaches.

This non-judgemental openness for alternative stories and the awareness that we are all shaped by our experiences is what a social constructionist supervisor would bring in order to fulfil this competency or standard.

Narrative practice talks about that practitioner having a de-centred but influential stance. The practitioner is fully there but not the centre. When the accreditation agencies standard and competency ask for the practitioner to use the "self" in the process, what they are referring to are situations in which the practitioner thinks that their own responses may be useful for the supervision client. An example may be that the supervisor had an experience very similar to that of the supervision client and they share it to ask the supervision client if that perspective evokes any awareness. Another example may be when the supervisor notices that a supervision client who is using a different coaching approach is describing something that the supervisor themselves would not engage with in a coaching session. The supervisor might then notice their own bias and either offer their alternative idea or not depending on the usefulness for the supervision client.

In this way the supervisor notices something about themselves, discerns whether this has something to offer for the supervision client or not, and when in doubt offers it to the supervision client without centring the supervisor. The same is true for other intuitions that the supervisor may have. Intuitions are based on our past experiences and they most often are embedded in the supervisor's experience and not necessarily in the supervision client's experience. However, sometimes they may be useful and can then be shared usefully.

Executes Professional Behaviours

A professional supervisor behaves professionally. What this means for the accreditation agencies is that a professional supervisor will inform their clients of standards of practice and reflect on how they are displaying the standards and competencies in their own practice, just like we are doing here in this chapter.

Part of professional behaviour is staying up to date and informed about current developments in the field. Building up and retaining credibility is not only important for the supervisor but also for the supervision clients. When the coaching supervisor is contracted by an organisation, and there is a double mandate to help with the development of the organisation's coaches and also help the organisation develop, the coaching supervisor will handle this double mandate ethically with a focus on value creation for all parties.

Some competencies of the accreditation agencies speak about the necessity of having "psychological knowledge". This is not described in detail, nor is it clear whether this refers specifically to knowledge of coaching psychology. The prescription of this as a necessity without sufficient specification places the burden on the coaching supervisor to decide whether to focus on this or not in coaching supervision. Solution Focused coaching supervision would not prescribe drawing on theoretical concepts but rather focusing on the sources of knowledge that the supervision client sees as relevant and useful.

Client and Client System

Solution Focused supervision operates on the premise that solutions are often more accessible and effective when individuals focus on their strengths and successes rather than on problems and deficits. In the context of coaching supervision, this approach extends its reach to not only address individual concerns but also to encompass the broader systemic dynamics at play within an organisation or team.

One key aspect of Solution Focused supervision that showcases its systemic awareness is its commitment to exploring and amplifying what is working well between people rather than inside people. Instead of dwelling on problems and obstacles, Solution Focused supervisors actively seek out instances of success and positive change. This approach fosters a mindset that acknowledges the interconnectedness of individuals within their interactional contexts, emphasising the ripple effects that positive changes can have on the entire organisation. By focusing on strengths and achievements, Solution Focused supervision inherently recognises the influence of systemic factors on individual and collective well-being. Furthermore, Solution Focused coaching supervision displays a keen awareness of human systems by promoting collaboration and co-creation. The supervisor acts as a facilitator, guiding individuals or teams to construct their own solutions by tapping into their unique strengths and resources. This collaborative process acknowledges the complexity of human systems, where diverse perspectives and contributions come together to shape the overall functioning of the organisation.

Another way in which Solution Focused coaching supervision showcases systemic awareness is through its focus on future-oriented thinking. Instead of dwelling on past mistakes or challenges, Solution Focused coaching supervision encourages individuals to envision and work towards a preferred future. This forward-focused approach acknowledges that human systems are dynamic and evolving entities, constantly influenced by the choices and actions of their members. By directing attention to future possibilities, Solution Focused coaching supervision aligns with the systemic understanding that change is an inherent and ongoing aspect of life. Solution Focused coaching supervision not only addresses individual concerns but also engages with the intricate web of relationships and interactions that characterise organisations. In so doing, Solution Focused coaching supervision offers a powerful and holistic approach that aligns with the complexities of human systems.

Facilitates Development of Supervision Client

Facilitating the development of the supervision client is the core purpose of coaching supervision. How Solution Focused coaching supervision encourages reflection and growth is described in the remainder of this book. A Solution Focused coaching supervisor's preference will be to invite the supervision client to develop their own ways of growing thereby centring the client. However, there may also be a point where the supervisor, as a more experienced practitioner, may be asked for advice and will then share it in a manner that promotes the autonomy of the supervision client.

Group Supervision

The ability to provide group supervision is another key competence mentioned by the accreditation agencies. In this book, we describe several structures that may be useful for group supervision. The accreditation agencies also mention that a coaching supervisor has the competence to "surface and manage group dynamics". Surfacing and managing group dynamics again positions the coaching supervisor outside the group in an observational position. In Solution Focus, we would translate that as: "the ability to co-construct useful conversations with the group". In our view it is not necessary to surface and manage group dynamics to do that. In a situation in which a group is not serving the purpose of helping the individual supervision group members to grow, the Solution Focused coaching supervisor would simply ask whether the group members are experiencing it similarly and what they would like instead from the coaching supervision and the coaching supervisor. Again, this exemplifies the Solution Focused stance of assuming that supervision clients are capable of co-creating learning and growth when provided with a conversational space to do so.

Reflective Exercise

In order to determine your own stance as a coaching supervisor, you may want to reflect on the following questions:

- What is your definition of coaching supervision?
- How do you demonstrate the core competencies/standards of a coaching supervisor?
- What are your coaching supervision clients noticing about you that tells them that you are demonstrating the core competencies?
- Take each competency/standard and think about great moments from your practice and not so great moments: what was the difference?

References

APECS (n.d.). *Ethical stance*. Retrieved February 6, 2024, from https://www.apecs.org/apecs-ethical-stance#guidelines

Association for Coaching (2018). *Coaching supervision guide*. https://cdn.ymaws.com/www.associationforcoaching.com/resource/resmgr/accreditation/coach_accreditation/supporting_documentation/ca_supervision_guide.pdf

Association of Coaching Supervisors (n.d.). *What is coaching supervision?* Retrieved February 6, 2024, from https://www.associationofcoachingsupervisors.com/supervisors/what-is-supervision#:~:text=is%20Coaching%20Supervision%3F-,What%20is%20Coaching%20Supervision%3F,the%20service%20of%20their%20clients.

Bachkirova, T. (2008). Coaching supervision: Reflection on changes and challenges. *People and Organisations at Work, Autumn*, 16–17.

Bachkirova, T., Jackson, P., Hennig, C. & Moral, M. (2020). Supervision in coaching: Systematic literature review. *International Coaching Psychology Review*, 15(2), 31–53. https://doi.org/10.53841/bpsicpr.2020.15.2.31.

Balint, E. (1985). The history of training and research in Balint groups. *Psychoanalytic Psychotherapy*, 1(2), 1–9. https://doi.org/10.1080/02668738500700111.

Belardi, N. (1994). *Supervision: Von der praxisberatung zur organisationsentwicklung* (*4th Ed*). Junfermann.

Carroll, M. (2007). Coaching psychology supervision: Necessity or luxury? In S. Palmer & A. Whybrow (Eds.). *Coaching psychology handbook*. Routledge.

Clutterbuck, D. (2022). *Coaching and mentoring. A journey through the models, theories, frameworks and narratives of David Clutterbuck* (*4th Ed*). Routledge.

De Shazer, S. (1984). The death of resistance. *Family Process*, 23(1), 1–17.

DGSv (2024). Historie. Retrieved February 6, 2024, from https://www.dgsv.de/der-verband/historie/

EMCC (2015). *Global code of ethics*. https://www.globalcodeofethics.org/download-the-code/

EMCC (2019). *EMCC supervision competency framework*. https://emccuk.org/common/Uploaded%20files/EMCC%20-%20competences%20-%20supervision%20-%20EN%20v2.pdf

Garvey, B. & Stokes, P. (2021). *Coaching and mentoring. Theory and practice* (*4th Ed*). SAGE.

Hawkins, P. & Shohet, R. (2012). *Supervision in the helping professions* (*4th Ed*). McGraw-Hill.

Hawkins, P. & Smith, N. (2006). *Coaching, mentoring and organizational consultancy: Supervision skills and development*. McGraw Hill Education.

ICF. (n.d.). *Coaching supervision*. Retrieved February 6, 2024, from *https://coach-ingfederation.org/credentials-and-standards/coaching-supervision*

ICF. (n.d.). Mentor Coaching. Retrieved February 6, 2024, from https://coach-ingfederation.org/credentials-and-standards/mentor-coaching

Inskipp, F. & Proctor, B. (1993). *The art, craft and tasks of counselling supervision. Professional development for counsellors, psychotherapists, supervisors and trainees – Pt. 1: Making the most of supervision (4th Ed)*. Cascade Publishing.

Kadushin, A. (1976). *Supervision in social work (1st Ed)*. Columbia University Press.

Lucas, M. & Larcombe, A. (2016). Helping independent coaches develop their business – A holistic approach to supervision or an opportunity for supervisors to exploit their position. *International Journal of Mentoring and Coaching, IX(3)*, 1–16.

Proctor, B. (1986). Supervision: A co-operative exercise in accountability. In M. Marken & M. Payne (Eds.). *Enabling and ensuring supervision in practice* (pp. 21–34). National Youth Bureau.

3 Solution Focused Coaching Supervision

Some Theory

Kirsten Dierolf

Introduction

Solution Focus is often labelled "the approach with no theory" and in some ways this is true in others not so much. So why this chapter? Theory is not like theory and like Ludwig Wittgenstein said: "The meaning of a word is its use in language" (Wittgenstein, 1958, p. 43). When we say that Solution Focus does not have "a theory", what we mean is that Solution Focused practitioners attempt to have as few theories **about their clients** as possible. They do not try to analyse internal dynamics of their clients, nor do they check whether the personality profile of their supervision client matches that of their customers or venture to notice and proclaim parallel processes as if they were a truth. In that sense, Solution Focused supervisors and other practitioners can live happily without theory.

However, that does not mean that Solution Focus does not have a theory about why we work in the way that we work or how we imagine our work will impact our clients positively. Solution Focused theory is understood as a way of distinguishing and explaining what we do and why it is quite thorough, and more thorough than many other coaching and supervision approaches. Solution Focused theory includes and is based on the epistemology and axiology of the approach. It is rooted deeply in social constructionist, post-structuralist and postmodern thought. In a world where many coaches and supervisors are attracted by the next new tool, the next new methodology and the next shiny new name, this is rather uncommon and maybe surprising. The implicit worldview of coaching approaches is very seldom uncovered, talked about or made transparent (Hurlow, 2022). It is possible to look at Solution Focus as merely a selection of tools and completely ignore the philosophical foundation at a practitioner level. A supervisor, however, who is asked to help supervision clients develop, needs a firm grounding in this kind of theory and needs to be aware of their own preferences and standpoint and how it may relate to the preferences and standpoints of their supervision clients.

In order to describe what makes the Solution Focused coaching supervision approach distinct in the space allotted in this book, we would like to revert to the Galveston declaration for conciseness and clarity purposes. The Galveston

DOI: 10.4324/9781003390527-3

declaration was one of the results of a conference in Galveston, Texas where Solution Focused, narrative and collaborative practitioners from various "helping" fields (therapy, coaching, social work) met to exchange knowledge and ideas. One working group started collaborating on the commonalities of these approaches and their discussion ended in the Galveston declaration (Gosnell et al., 2017).

The Galveston declaration was developed in a format that resembles the Agile Manifesto (Beck et al., 2001). In keeping with the social constructionist preference for acknowledging different perspectives rather than proclaiming singular valid truth, the Galveston declaration does not proclaim that social constructionist approaches are "true" or "better". Instead, the declaration is framed according to what practitioners value more over what they value less. In the following we would like to walk you through the value statements of the Galveston declaration and make connections to what this means for Solution Focused supervision. We hope that it will become clear how Solution Focused supervision is different from other approaches and why it chooses to engage in some practices and not in others. Another hope is that the reader might reflect on their own value statements and preferences in light of the ones mentioned below (Table 3.1).

Table 3.1 Declaration of Values

We Value This	More Than This
PLURALISM – differences of view	**SINGULARITY – of view**
1. Acknowledging multiple "truths"	1. Holding to a singular firm belief
2. Responsiveness to particularities in context	2. Applying generalities (including diagnosis)
3. Exploring multiple social realities	3. Searching for a single reality
4. Exploring multiple cultures, contexts, and interactions, and influences	4. Privileging specific cultures over others
FLUX – differences of state	**STATIC – fixed states**
1. Facilitating the emergence of new identities	1. Stabilizing fixed or rigid identity/ identities
2. Regarding "every interaction as mutual influence" with potential for unidirectional influence	2. Assuming "neutrality and objectivity"
3. Recognizng people as persons embedded in relationships	3. Treating people as separate individuals
4. Experimenting with transformational restorative justice practices	4. Implementing traditional retributive justice practices
OPENING SPACE – expanding choice	**CLOSING SPACE – removing choice**
1. Living with curiosity	1. Living with certainty
2. Opening space for enlivened possibilities	2. Closing space for problems to persist

(Continued)

Table 3.1 (Continued)

We Value This	More Than This
3. Inviting others to entertain change	3. Imposing change interventions upon others
4. Proactively including others (while respecting their possible choice to remain apart)	4. Passively and/or actively excluding others from participating
RESPONSIBILITY – generativity	**DEFICIT FOCUS – constraint**
1. Noticing resources, competencies, and possibilities	1. Identifying and diagnosing deficits, dysfunctions, and limitations for correction
2. Anticipating potential effects of resource use and developing sustainable ecologies	2. Utilizing profitable resources without consideration of the consequences
3. Assuming collective responsibility	3. Projecting responsibility and specifying to whom it belongs; judging others
4. Enacting an ethics of caring and privileging restorative justice	4. Applying moral judgements and retributive justice

Source: Gosnell et al. (2017, p. 25).

The Galveston Declaration

We Value Pluralism – Differences of View More Than Singularity of View

We Value Acknowledging Multiple "Truths" More Than Holding to a Singular Firm Belief

Solution Focus is a postmodern, post-structuralist and social construction-ist approach. One of the positions held by these approaches is that whatever can be said is always said from the vantage point of someone and that there is no "neutrality" or "objectivity". Postmodern, post-structuralist and social constructionist philosophies worry less about what is real and not real and more about the social realities in which what counts as real is constructed. The fundamental view of a person is less of a mind which is separated from its environment and more of a person who is always in the process of being shaped by their environment and shaping their environment at the same time. It's not about a differentiation between a knowing subject and the known world but more about the interactions of the person with the world and with themselves. These ontological and epistemological positions are the reasons why acknowledging multiple truths is valued by and inevitable for postmodern, post-structuralist and social constructionist approaches.

For Solution Focused supervision this means that supervisor will strive to co-construct useful interactions with the supervision client. They will acknowledge that neither supervisor nor supervision client has privileged access to what is right or true. The intention of the supervision session is to create interactions which fulfil the purposes of coaching supervision: restorative, developmental and quality assuring.

The supervision client is not viewed as an object of analysis by the supervisor. In fact, having this outside view of other human beings (as if this was possible) is frowned upon or even deemed unethical. Treating human beings as "knowable" objects is not appropriate. Postmodern approaches are sometimes criticised as "relativist". We don't think this is true as valuing equality of human beings is one of the fundamental principles – any position which rejects the fundamental idea of equality would necessarily be outside the framework.

For the supervision session, this means that neither the worldview of the supervision client nor the worldview of the supervisor is privileged. The supervision client is centred in the conversation and can explore their topics and the supervisor is also there fully as a human being with their own views which may helpfully serve to broaden the perspective of the supervision client but not as a truth which the supervision client needs to accept about themselves.

We Value Responsiveness to Particularities in Context More Than
Applying Generalities (Including Diagnosis)

The focus in Solution Focused coaching supervision is the further development of the supervision client. This may be stating the obvious, but there are approaches to coach supervision in which the focus of the discussion is "what is **really** going on with the client of the coaching supervision client". We don't want to sound polemical here, but most of the authors of this book have experienced such coaching supervision. The supervision clients speak about their cases and the supervisors will attempt to provide a "diagnosis" for the supervision client's client. Diagnoses we have heard are "probably an alcoholic" or "a narcissist" from psychologically trained supervisors, "typically orange level" by Integral coaching supervisors or "a very strong red" by Insights Discovery practitioners. This may seem helpful at first as it suggests a "right" way forward: the "real" problem was identified, a fitting framework found and a standard solution applied. You can probably see why this does not fit with the above-mentioned viewpoint. Human interactions are complex, and it is impossible to identify clear pathways or cause and effect relationships. Dave Snowden describes his "Cynefin" framework: In "complex systems [...] causal relationships are entangled and dynamic and the only way to understand the system is to interact with it" (Greenberg & Bertsch, 2022, p. 18). Solution Focused coaching supervisors therefore refrain from "diagnosing" coaching clients or using a fixed framework to guide supervision clients' behaviours. Both of these behaviours would mean that the coaching supervisor takes an "outside the system" position which is neither possible nor helpful. With the awareness of the complexity of the supervision client's interactions with the supervisor (and the client), the Solution Focused coaching supervisor will not provide cookie cutter solutions for what needs to be done with the supervision client's client but will invite the coaching supervision client to describe and explore what their preferred outcome is and what ways of interacting with the supervision client's client fit with the current and preferred future identity of the coaching supervision client.

Solution Focused supervision is therefore about the coaching supervision client and not about the clients of the coaching supervision client. The clients are not there, there is nothing that we can do about the client in the session – Solution Focused supervisors focus on the interaction between coaching supervisor and supervision client. In this way, the focus is on what the supervision client has agency over versus extrapolating what the supervision client's client was thinking, or might do, which the supervision client can neither validate nor comment on. This could lead to the supervision client implementing suggestions based on the input from the supervisor "on the client" and inadvertently backfire.

Another distinction that can be made is that Solution Focused supervision also refrains from "diagnosing" the supervision client and their development as a coach. The frameworks that are sometimes used come from adult development theory (Kegan, 1982), from spiral dynamics which has again become popular through the works of Frederic Laloux (2014), the various personality tests or from the competence frameworks of the international coaching organisations: ICF (2018), EMCC (2015) and AC (2012). All of these have in common that they suggest a standard development path for any coach from "foundation" to "mastery level" with "competency frameworks that are as yet unsubstantiated" (Bachkirova & Smith, 2015, p. 127).

In "Theory of Solution Focused Practice", a collaboration of several prominent Solution Focused experts from various fields published by the European Brief Therapy Association in 2020 we read: "Solution-focused practice doesn't have a theory of development of its own. Instead, when needed for the change at hand, it uses the theories individual clients find useful" (Sundman et al., 2020). In practice, Solution Focused coaching supervisors work with clients from various coaching approaches. If the client has a developmental framework and likes working with it, the Solution Focused coaching supervisor will respect the client's worldview and preferences while at the same time being aware of the limitations that such frameworks might entail. As Tom Strong, Karen H. Ross and Monica Sesma Vazques phrase it: "[…] humans are best served by being able to judiciously draw on the resources of multiple discourses, and that problems can emerge when they overcommit to the resources of a single discourse" (Strong et al., 2015, p. 4). The Solution Focused coaching supervisor will not privilege their own Solution Focused worldview over their client but also invite the client to consider moving beyond totalising discourses about themselves or their own clients.

This is also the reason why there is no "standard formula", model or framework that guides a Solution Focused coaching supervision session, like, for example, the seven-eyed model of Peter Hawkins and colleagues (2020, pp. 87–88) that suggests helpful areas the supervisor might focus on. The content and process are co-created and not driven by the supervisor's analysis, selection of focus or identification of a fitting "intervention". We don't think that many other approaches still work with a model of the "expert supervisor" who "analyses" the supervision client and don't want to create a strawman. However, the distinction is gradual and Solution Focused coaching supervision is radical in its focus on the interaction and co-creation between supervisor and supervision client.

We Value Exploring Multiple Social Realities More Than Searching for a Single Reality

As we value pluralism rather than singularity of view it follows that exploring multiple social realities is preferred over searching for a single reality. Supervision clients may come with their stories about an event or about their current or preferred identity as a coach. Searching for a single reality in supervision may be tied to finding a singular explanation for what happened or for who the coaching supervision client is. For example, a coaching supervision client might be distraught about not having been able to help a coaching client solve a problem and feel incapable as a coach. Searching for a single reality, an explanation might invite the supervision client to look for past experiences of despair or feeling like a failure to resolve the "trauma". By understanding that these past events are "causing" the emotional "overreaction" now, the supervision client might differentiate the past from the present and come to a different view of themselves (hopefully as capable and able to learn). While the outcome may be helpful and create relief for the supervision client, this kind of coaching supervision is looking for an explanation, a single reality.

Solution Focused supervision values exploring multiple social realities. To quote a book title from narrative therapy: We want to invite our clients to tell their stories in ways that makes them stronger (Wingard & Lester, 2001). We are aware that there are always multiple stories that can be told about any event and invite descriptions rather than explanations (McKergow, 2021, pp. 62–63). Rather than figuring out why the supervision client is feeling a sense of failure, a Solution Focused supervisor would invite the supervision client to describe what they want instead and how that might play out in their social realities: "Suppose you felt more … how would you notice, what would others notice, how would you respond etc." (read more in our sections on Supervision Moves in Chapter 4, p. 42). If the supervision client wants to find an explanation and make their own sense of what happened, we would invite making "sense of the world in order so we can act in it", as Dave Snowden (2022, p. 64) puts it. Rather than figuring out a correct explanation, a simple causal relation, we assume that human relationships are complex, and making sufficient sense to act is all we can do. Paul Cilliers called this a "modest position" – we know that we don't know for sure, but that does not mean we cannot say anything (Cilliers, 2005). In the linear-causality paradigm, it is a common stated desire that people want to understand and know why something occurred. Traditional approaches often focus on this, leading to interpretations and labels. Solution Focused supervisors would respond differently to this never-ending cycle of exploring "the why" by being curious about the desire behind the need to know. The understanding of the "why" is a route to something beyond the question, and this often leads to responses like, "Then I can move on" or "Then I will feel confident about what to do". Our questions bypass the assumption that insight or understanding must occur before change can happen. However, insight often is a by-product after inviting the supervision client to "Imagine you know all you need to know about 'why'. What difference would this make?"

We Value Exploring Multiple Cultures, Contexts, and Interactions, and Influences More Than Privileging Specific Cultures over Others

Coaching supervision clients come from various contexts. In the globalised world of online coaching and supervision both supervisors and coaches are navigating multiple cultures daily. Each of these cultures has different local norms of correctness and distributions of rights and duties. We don't only mean national cultures, but the many contexts supervisors and supervision clients are faced with: the culture of their organisations, the culture within their coaching community and approach and the culture of the clients that they serve (for example, business or life coaching). The Solution Focused coaching supervisor intends to support their clients to work within their context and approach and does not privilege their own culture, context and approach. The specific context of the supervision client is always in view, for example, through perspective change questions: "Suppose you … how would your client notice?" This way, Solution Focused coaching supervisors can act helpfully for coaches from various contexts and with various approaches (for more detail, see Chapter 7 on "Coaching Supervision with Clients Using Different Coaching Models/Approaches").

Our awareness of multiple contexts and cultures also allows us to invite supervision clients to explore the dominant narratives within their contexts and determine the relationship they would like to have with them: do they agree, do they want to resist and do they want to integrate? For example, a supervision client might bring a case where they are trying to support a female executive in her new role. The supervisor notices how the client is struggling to balance family life and the demands of their new position. The client may have very high demands on herself, and the supervision client might feel bad about supporting these, in their view, overly high demands. The supervisor might then explore with the supervision client what they might call that narrative, which relationship they personally would want with it and how this relationship might positively influence their relationship with their client and help the client (or not).

We Value Flux – Differences of State More Than Static – Fixed States

We Value Facilitating the Emergence of New Identities More Than Stabilising Fixed or Rigid Identity/Identities

As stated above stabilising fixed or rigid identity/identities by "diagnoses" or fixed frameworks is not something Solution Focused supervisors find helpful unless this is a framework the supervision client brings and is working with. One of the aims of Solution Focused supervision is to expand the number of choices for the supervision client. We would invite changing perspectives and gently (with permission) challenge fixed or rigid views of the supervision client about themselves or their clients. Of course, this would only ever be invitational and not confrontational, a "tap on the shoulder" (Thomas, 2013, p. 127) rather than advice given with the assumption that the supervisor is "right".

Kirsten once had a coaching supervision client whose client did not appreciate the methodology she was using. The supervision client was using Solution Focused coaching while the client wanted to explore "her inner obstacles to what she wants to achieve". Inviting the supervision client to soften her identity as a Solution Focused coach and allowing her to find out ways in which she could stay true to what was important to her (focusing on resources and progress) and still serve the client without inviting her to resist the methodology by insisting on it was very helpful.

We Value Regarding "Every Interaction as Mutual Influence" With Potential for Unidirectional Influence More Than Assuming "Neutrality and Objectivity"

There is no human interaction that does not leave both parties unchanged. As stated above we prefer to think of ourselves as collaborating and co-creating with our supervision clients rather than pretending to be "neutral observers". We value a real, caring and flexible relationship with the supervision clients and aim to show up as the people we are. Of course, the supervision client is in the centre of the conversation – it is about what they want to achieve and who they are and not about the supervisor's goals or reality. Michael White coined the term "decentred but influential" for the position of a narrative practitioner (Gaddis, 2016). This is the same in Solution Focused supervision.

Solution Focused supervision focuses on the interaction between coaching supervisor and supervision client (and not on the supervision client's client nor an analysis of the supervision client). The Solution Focused supervisor will therefore do their best to collaborate usefully with the respective supervision client and how they like to learn, develop, experience restoration from potentially difficult situations. Each supervision client is unique. Solution Focused supervisors need to be experts in creating a collaborative space. There is no given structure or format that is used every time, only a preference for focusing on what is wanted and what is already working. The whole supervision session is emergent: if it were a dance, it would not be a choreographed one, but one like the Lindy Hop or Tango Argentino where the moves are created in response to the other dancer and not pre-planned in advance.

We Value Recognising People as Persons Embedded in Relationships
More Than Treating People as Separate Individuals

No supervision happens in a vacuum. Coaching supervision clients work with clients, with client organisations, with coaching providers, with their own team (if they are internal coaches) and so on. Solution Focused supervision will always assume that there are important relationships and interactions in the supervision client's life that can be drawn into the coaching supervision conversation, as recounted by the client. They can also be raised in other ways. The coaching supervision client might engage in "feedback informed coaching" where they ask their clients for feedback to improve their coaching (Miller et al., 2020). The coaching supervision client and coaching supervisor might have a conversation with the coach's organisation (if they are an internal coach). The coaching supervisor and supervision client might listen to a recording of an actual coaching session together. We would acknowledge all perspectives but ultimately know that we are working with the coaching supervision client's account of their experience and privilege their sense making in the context of their daily interactions.

We Value Experimenting With Transformational Restorative Justice Practices
More Than Implementing Traditional Retributive Justice Practices

Sometimes coaching supervision is about quality insurance. Frank Thomas (2013, pp. 110–114) talks about the "Indirect-Direct Communication" spectrum in supervision: Metaphor, Semaphore and Two-by-Four. Metaphor is about ambiguous communication which the supervision makes sense of, stories, questions and so on. Semaphore is more direct communication in which the supervisor provides guidance and the "Two-by-Four" is a whack on the head. Now, that does not sound like a preference for "restorative justice". However, as direct as a Solution Focused coaching supervisor may be, for example in the case of an ethical violation, the goal will always be to find better ways in the future. This is best done without blame and negative character judgements about the coaching supervision client. We assume that each coaching supervision client did the best they could with the information that they had at the time: brainstorming beats blamestorming.

If a client of our supervision client came to any harm due to the actions of the supervision client, a Solution Focused supervisor would aim at encouraging the supervision client to "make it right", to talk to the client, apologise or do whatever it takes to restore the relationship. You can read more on this in Chapter 5 on ethics.

We Value Opening Space – Expanding Choice More Than Closing Space – Removing Choice

We Value Living With Curiosity More Than Living with Certainty

Curiosity is very important for coaching supervisors. A curious stance in the supervision process will lead the supervisor to ask questions and to listen closely to what the supervision client is sharing. In Solution Focused coaching supervision, the supervisor attempts to tune into the language of the supervision client – using the supervision client's words and inviting the supervision client to explore important words.

The supervisor may suspect that some language the client uses carries more importance than other language. For example: "I woke up at eight today" might be less meaningful than "I was so touched by the candour of my client". The key word here is "might" – even when picking up language that seems important, the coaching supervisor remains curious and in a "not-knowing" stance. They may pick up what seems important **to them** but always check with the supervision client whether this really is something important and that they would like to explore it. After all, "waking up at eight" might be a great breakthrough and "being touched by the candour of the client" something that happens daily and may be nothing special to explore.

This curiosity and related "not-knowing" stance is also reflected in the language Solution Focused supervisors use: tentative and presuppositional. Tentative language is used to leave the creation of meaning and focus to the supervision client. The supervisor's language also presupposes that the supervision client is resourceful and whole, that they have strengths and good intentions. A question like "How did you know to respond this way?", for example, presupposes that the supervision client knows something and has some experience. "Suppose you develop your skill of listening even further, what difference would that make" presupposes that the supervision client has listening skills, that they can be developed further and that this might make a (positive) difference.

Creating a supervision agreement with the supervision client is another place where the Solution Focused supervisor will stay curious throughout the session. As we know that conversations and thoughts are emergent, the agreement that was mentioned in the beginning of a session may not be what the client walks away with. This is not a mistake – it just sometimes happens that directions shift. The Solution Focused supervisor will be curious about these shifts and the options and choices they provide rather than shutting down a potentially interesting discussion because it does not fit with the original agreement.

We Value Opening Space for Enlivened Possibilities More Than Closing Space for Problems to Persist

In Solution Focus, we assume that change always happens and that it makes sense to identify changes that already are going into the right direction. This is one way of "opening space for enlivened possibilities". Another way of opening space for possibilities in supervision is to invite the client to describe what is wanted rather than what is not wanted and what is already working rather than what is not working.

Sometimes, Solution Focus is misunderstood – the name suggests a narrowing of the focus solely on "Solutions" as if nothing else is important or can be talked about in a Solution Focused session, be it coaching, therapy or supervision. Of course, the client can talk about anything they want to talk about. The practitioner will collaborate, listen for what is wanted, listen for what is working and invite the client to describe this. If the client wants to talk about what they think is problematic, not wanted and not working, the practitioner will obviously listen – anything else is not respectful and would not centre the client but the practitioner's view of what should happen.

We sometimes use the image of a "coaching house" which could equally be a "supervision house" or a "Solution Focused Practice" house. We imagine what is problematic and not working as happening in the basement. There are a few questions that may help to invite moving to the first or ground floor: "What would you like instead?", "What difference would that make?", "How are you coping so far?", "When was there a time when things were different?"

We Value Inviting Others to Entertain Change More Than
Imposing Change Interventions Upon Others

Imposing change interventions upon others is difficult for two reasons, one practical, the other more theoretical. Supervisors who think in term of "interventions" possibly mistake human interactions as predictable – complicated rather than complex (Snowden, 2022). If you believe a "change intervention" can be successfully "imposed" on others, you must be confident that your intervention will have the desired results. However, human beings are not trivial machines where the same input will always have the same output – so any action of the supervisor will always have to respond to the situation at hand, be tentative, and an experiment with an uncertain outcome rather than an "intervention". The more practical reason is that people do not like being imposed on. Supervision clients are much more likely to implement changes that they developed themselves. Also these changes are probably more fitting to the supervision client's context, since the supervision client knows their context much better than the supervisor can. Even in situations in which the supervisor feels they have to give strong guidance, asking the supervision client for their input and stance towards the guidance seems more promising than simply telling people what to do.

We Value Proactively Including Others (While Respecting Their Possible Choice
to Remain Apart) More Than Passively and/or Actively Excluding Others
From Participating

Solution Focused group and individual supervision will be a voluntary activity. If someone does not want to join, the supervisor will explore what would need to happen, so that the client would feel that this is a useful activity. On the other hand, the Solution Focused group or team supervisor will take care to include anyone who may be interested in the result of the supervision in the supervision.

We Value Responsibility – Generativity More Than Deficit Focus – Constraint

We Value Noticing Resources, Competencies, and Possibilities More Than Identifying and Diagnosing Deficits, Dysfunctions, and Limitations for Correction

As the Solution Focused supervisor focuses on what is wanted and what is working, it is only natural that noticing resources, competencies and possibilities is preferred. Paying attention to what the supervision client is doing well and amplifying that, has the additional advantage that the successes of the supervision client happened in their context and are likely fitting that context. Often supervision clients attribute their successes to their clients – coaches seem to be a humble bunch. Of course, they value their clients and attribute a lot of what went well to what their clients did (and probably rightfully so). In Solution Focused coaching supervision, the supervisor will ask about the agency of the supervision client: What did they do to help their clients be successful? Becoming aware of what the supervision client did that might have been helpful makes it repeatable and turns it into a conscious competence.

Another useful place to look when discussing a problem, a lack of competence or something that did not go well is "unique outcomes" or "exceptions". When it was better, what did the supervision client do differently? Again, these "unique outcomes" or "exceptions" happened in the supervision client's context and describing them might bring up useful ideas for actions.

The assumption is always that the supervision client tried their best with the knowledge that they had at the time, however negatively they might be evaluating the situation in hindsight. As we know, this is always 20/20. Supervision is an activity geared towards reflection, learning and development – being afraid of mistakes, beating oneself up or becoming defensive are all not conducive to that.

We Value Anticipating Potential Effects of Resource Use and Developing Sustainable Ecologies More Than Utilising Profitable Resources Without Consideration of the Consequences

We live in a critical age where what we do today may have consequences for many generations to come. Considering the consequences of our actions for the human and non-human environment is important for any human activity these days. Solution Focused supervision invites clients to reflect on the consequences of their actions on their context by inviting them to change their perspective: what will others notice when they act in a certain way, how would they respond and so on?

We Value Assuming Collective Responsibility More Than Projecting Responsibility and Specifying and Accountability to Whom It Belongs; Judging Others

Any action happens in a context, an environment, a community or culture with differing ways of gauging what is ethical or correct. Nobody makes decisions solely on their own. As Rom Harré said in an interview with Kirsten Dierolf: "Thinking, denoting, reasoning, deciding are all primarily interactions rather than personal actions. They may look like personal actions but when you do a thorough study of how they operate you find they are ultimately basically interactions" (Dierolf, 2012, p. 80). It is therefore neither fair nor useful to "blame" the individual supervision client when something went wrong, or an "unethical" decision was taken. It is the responsibility of the supervisor to ensure that something is learned, this will not happen again and that some form of restorative justice takes place if someone was hurt in any way. Punishing or shaming the supervision client is rarely conducive to fulfilling this responsibility.

The stance of the supervisor is more "*insert favorite expletive* – that wasn't good. How can I help my supervision client get out of this mess and learn from it and what are the contextual factors or narratives that might have contributed to this?" rather than judging the client. Often, the environment can also help to prevent unfortunate events in coaching. Kirsten once supervised a coach who had inadvertently breached confidentiality by disclosing more information to the sponsor than the client had agreed would be shared. One of the solutions of the coach was to take care only to have three-way conversations with client and sponsor present – a shift in the environment rather than in the coach.

By not judging or blaming, the Solution Focused supervisor also collaborates better with the supervision client and flattens hierarchy. This way, coaching supervision can be a collaborative journey of exploration.

We Value Enacting an Ethics of Caring and Privileging Restorative Justice More Than Applying Moral Judgements and Retributive Justice

This ties in very neatly with what was mentioned above: caring and restorative justice rather than blame and punishment. Blame and punishment are the best antidotes for learning – that's why we don't go there. The blame frame is demoralising and does not promote exploration of change. Bringing a person gently and respectfully to integrating what they have learned is a kind of resilience training. Finding meaning and utilising opportunities to learn and grow facilitates healthy growth.

Reflective Exercise

- Take the Galveston declaration, just the main points or the main points and the sub-points and reflect on whether you would like to take them on-board, edit or reject them in any way for your practice.
- Formulate your own adaptations.
- Think of practical applications – where does what you value show up in your supervision practice (or if you are new to supervision, how would you like it to show up in your practice?)
- You might also use your reflections to start writing a "personal statement" about your thinking and approach to supervision (which is also required by European Mentoring and Coaching Council (EMCC) should you wish to become accredited as a coaching supervisor).

References

Association for Coaching (2012). *AC Coaching Competency Framework*. https://cdn.ymaws.com/www.associationforcoaching.com/resource/resmgr/Accreditation/Accred_General/Coaching_Competency_Framewor.pdf

Bachkirova, T. & Smith, C.L. (2015). From competencies to capabilities in the assessment and accreditation of coaches. *International Journal of Evidence Based Coaching and Mentoring 13*(2), 123–140.

Beck, K., Beedle, M., van Bennekum, A., Cockburn, A., Cunningham, W., Fowler, M., Grenning, J., Highsmith, J., Hunt, A., Jeffries, R., Kern, J., Marick, B., Martin, R.C., Mellor, S., Schwaber, K., Sutherland, J. & Thomas, D. (2001). *The agile manifesto*. https://agilemanifesto.org/

Cilliers, P. (2005). Complexity, deconstruction and relativism. *Theory, Culture & Society 22*(5), 255–267.

Dierolf, K. (2012). Rom Harré: The new psychology — Discursive practices not internal forces. *InterAction 4*(2), 78–86.

EMCC (2015). EMCC Competence Framework. https://www.emccglobal.org/wp-content/uploads/2018/10/EMCC-competences-framework-v2-EN.pdf

Gaddis, S. (2016). Poststructural inquiry: Narrative therapy's de-centered and influential stance. In V.C. Dickerson (Ed.) *Poststructural and narrative thinking in family therapy* (pp. 9–27). Springer.

Gosnell, F., McKergow, M., Moore, B., Mudry, T. & Tomm, K. (2017) A Galveston declaration. *Journal of Systemic Therapies 36*(3), 20–26. https://doi.org/10.1521/jsyt.2017.36.3.20.

Greenberg, R. & Bertsch, B. (Ed.) (2022). *Cynefin (R). Weaving sense-making into the fabric of our world* (2nd ed). Cognitive Edge.

Hawkins, P., McMahon, A., Ryde, J. & Wilmot, J. (2020). *Supervision in the helping professions* (5th ed). Open University Press.

Hurlow, S. (2022). Revisiting the relationship between coaching and learning: The problems and possibilities. *Academy of Management and Learning Education 21*(1), 121–138. https://doi.org/10.5465/amle.2019.0345.

International Coaching Federation (2018). *ICF core competencies*. Retrieved 4 February, 2023, from https://coachingfederation.org/credentials-and-standards/core-competencies.

Kegan, R. (1982). *The evolving self: Problem and process in human development*. Harvard University Press.

Laloux, F. (2014). *Reinventing organisations. A guide to creating organisations inspired by the next stage in human consciousness.* Nelson Parker.

McKergow, M. (2021). *The next generation of solution focused practice. Stretching the world for new opportunities and progress.* Routledge.

Miller, S.D., Hubble, M.A. & Chow, D. (2020). *Better results. Using deliberate practice to improve therapeutic effectiveness.* American Psychological Association.

Snowden, D. (2022). Cynefin in brief. In R. Greenberg and B. Bertsch (Eds.) *Cynefin (R). Weaving sense-making into the fabric of our world* (2nd ed), pp. 64–69. Cognitive Edge.

Strong, T., Ross, K.H. & Sesma-Vazquez, M. (2015). Counselling the (self?) Diagnosed client: Generative and reflective conversations. *British Journal of Guidance & Counselling 43*(5), 598–610. https://doi.org/10.1080/03069885.2014.996736.

Sundman, P., Schwab, M., Wolf, F., Wheeler, J., Cabié, M., van der Hoorn, S., Pakrosnis, R., Dierolf, K. & Hjerth, M. (2020). *Theory of solution-focused practice. Version 2020.* Books on Demand.

Thomas, F.N. (2013). *Solution-focused supervision.* Springer.

Wingard, B. & Lester, J. (2001). *Telling our stories in ways that make us stronger* (2nd ed). Dulwich Centre Publications.

Wittgenstein, L. (1958, 2001). *Philosophical investigations: The German text*, with a Revised English Translation 50th Anniversary Commemorative Edition. Wiley.

4 Individual Solution Focused Coaching Supervision

Kirsten Dierolf and Debbie Hogan

Introduction

In this chapter we outline the coaching supervision "moves" a Solution Focused (SF) coaching supervisor can use during a supervision session. The metaphor of the "Art Gallery Walk" which provides a possible useful structure for a supervision session is explored. Other "moves" of the supervisor and the client are described as per function of the coaching supervision. Some concrete examples are provided for how SF supervisors might respond when called to provide assistance in one of the supervisory functions.

The Gallery

The idea of using the metaphor of a "gallery" for SF practice comes from BRIEF in London and has been written about by Mark McKergow (2021). The metaphor likens a SF session, be it coaching, therapy, counselling or supervision to a visit to an art gallery. We first enter the ticket office – if you don't have a ticket, you cannot get in. This is the contracting phase of the session. The other two rooms are the "preferred future gallery", which is about a rich description of what the client would like, and the "successful past gallery" where the practitioner will invite the client to describe instances of their preferred future which are already happening in the present. The last room is the "gift shop" where the practitioner and client discuss what the client will be taking away. In Figure 4.1 is an image of such a gallery as it relates to supervision.

In the following, we would like to describe the four different rooms in more detail.

Ticket Office

As in coaching, also in coaching supervision, we have two ticket offices: one ticket office where supervisor and supervision client create "the ticket" for the whole supervision process and one for each session.

"The ticket" for the whole supervision process is created in the first session of several supervision sessions. The supervisor invites the coaching

DOI: 10.4324/9781003390527-4

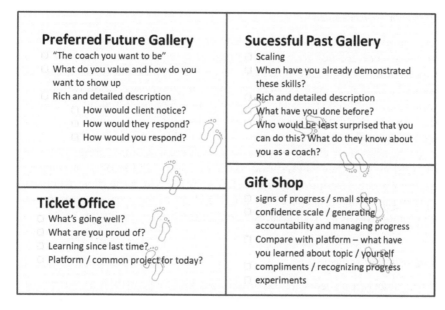

Preferred Future Gallery
"The coach you want to be"
What do you value and how do you
want to show up
Rich and detailed description
    How would client notice?
    How would they respond?
    How would you respond?

Sucessful Past Gallery
Scaling
When have you already demonstrated
these skills?
Rich and detailed description
What have you done before?
Who would be least surprised that you
can do this? What do they know about
you as a coach?

Ticket Office
What's going well?
What are you proud of?
Learning since last time?
Platform / common project for today?

Gift Shop
signs of progress / small steps
confidence scale / generating
accountability and managing progress
Compare with platform – what have
you learned about topic / yourself
compliments / recognizing progress
experiments

Figure 4.1 The Solution Focused art gallery
(Image by Kirsten Dierolf)

supervision client to describe what will be different after the whole supervision process. They begin with the end in mind. In SF coaching, the client usually determines when the coaching process ends. This may be different in coaching supervision. Coaching supervision often has its own rhythm. For example, European Mentoring and Coaching Council (EMCC) requires every coach to take a supervision session every quarter or for every 35 hours of coaching practice. Also coaching platforms or companies that the coach is working for may require regular coaching supervision. This means that there is not a natural end in sight. Nevertheless, a SF supervisor and their client will agree desired outcomes for a period of time that seems logical.

The "session ticket office" is the space in which the supervision client and supervisor agree on what is going to happen in this session, what the ideal outcome of this session may be and how the session is going to run. The supervisor might mention the functions of supervision and ask the client to choose the function that would serve them best at this moment: restorative, quality insurance or ethical considerations, for example. Once both supervisor and client are clear on and the best hopes of the client for the outcome of the session, know the function that the supervision should have and how the supervision should best be run, they can start moving to the other parts of the gallery.

Preferred Future Gallery

The gallery model seems like a predetermined path. However, the rooms of the gallery are not to be understood as a sequence that happens all the time. The supervisor and supervision client move back and forth through the rooms, and it may even be possible that the supervision session has several topics and that each step is taken several times. The preferred future gallery is the space in which the client is invited to describe the outcome that they are seeking from the supervision session in observable details: who they will be as a coach, what their clients or other stakeholders will notice about them after the session, how they will respond to their response and so on. The purpose is to create a rich description of the preferred future which the client will be able to recognise when it happens. Inviting the client to focus on signs of improvement and growth by itself creates a pool in the desired direction.

Successful Past Gallery

When supervision clients are looking for any kind of growth, it is a growth that they can imagine. We don't think that it is possible to imagine something if you don't have any experience of this or something similar ever happening to you. If there is a wish, there usually also are experiences which can be used as resources. We sometimes refer to this as the "resourceful past". We've described in other chapters how this is a kind of resource activation. For example, if the supervision client would like to act more in partnership with their clients, they probably have an idea what this would look like. In SF supervision, the supervisor would invite the supervision client to explore in great detail those instances in which they were already able to partner with their clients at least a little bit. That way the supervision client becomes even clearer on what it is that they would like to achieve. By being aware of how they partner with their clients, a supervision client also is able to notice more clearly when they are already doing it, and subsequently do more of what works for them. With the exploration of the precedent they also become more hopeful that they can develop the skill that they would like to develop. Supervision moves used in SF supervision that serve this purpose include scaling or asking for instances of the desired future already happening.

Gift Shop

In every museum you have the gift shop in which the visitors to the museums are invited to buy delightful things that they can take away to remind them of their visit. In SF supervision sessions, the client, too, is invited to think about what they are going to be taking away. The preference here is for asking the client what they would notice in their practice after the session that would tell them that they are getting better at what they want to improve or develop. We also invite supervision clients to think about what their clients might be noticing about them. The idea is to come up with concrete descriptions of observable behaviour and the impact of that change on others. Usually supervision clients will come up with experiments around moving forward with the goal with which they entered the supervision session or which they developed in the supervision session.

Here is an example highlighting how the supervisor invites the supervision client to describe what they will be taking from the supervision that supports the change they want to see in their development as a coach.

Coaching supervisor:	You mentioned earlier that you wanted to have more confidence in coaching senior executives, especially those who work in a context you're not familiar with. So, what are you hoping to take with you by the end of our session that will tell you that exploring this was helpful?
Coaching supervision client:	Well, I guess if I had some ideas about how to manage my anxiety and some ideas about being calm and present during the coaching so I can really listen, that would help.
Coaching supervisor:	So, some ideas about managing your anxiety and ideas about being calm and present, so you can really listen. You'd know it was useful if you had some ideas around that?
Coaching supervision client:	Yes! Well, I guess I already do some of that and know a little bit about that since I practice meditation and I've been working on that.
Coaching supervisor:	Ok, sure. You already know some things and have done some things to have more confidence. Would it be helpful to start with what you're already doing or do you want to go somewhere else?
Coaching supervision client:	Actually, just now I'm realising I do practice some things to help me be more confident, but I don't feel that is enough.
Coaching supervisor:	So, you've already got some ideas to improve your confidence and you want to explore more, is that right?
Coaching supervision client:	Yes, that would be really helpful.
Coaching supervisor:	So, just to be clear, you're hoping by the end of the session to take some ideas, old and new ones to help you with your confidence.
Coaching supervision client:	Yes …
Coaching supervisor:	Ok, so at the end of our coaching, we can circle back to this to see if the ideas that have emerged are sufficient for helping you have more confidence in coach executives.

Supervision Moves

Allow us to switch metaphors. We are no longer in the art gallery or museum but we're on the dance floor. In keeping with the social constructionist idea that all communication is co-creation, a SF supervisor will not think in terms of tools or techniques to be used on a supervision client. A more apt metaphor is that of moves on the dance floor in which supervisor and supervision client respond to one another and co-create learning. In the following you will find some standard "dance moves" of SF supervisors. Please remember that these are not moves that happen in every session or that follow a strategic agenda or standard decision tree. They are part of the repertoire of the SF supervisor and they may happen in an SF supervision session. However, there might be SF supervision sessions in which none of these appear. What makes a supervision SF is a focus on progress and resources in whichever way that focus can be co-created between supervisor and supervision client and not an array of standard strategies or tools.

We have ordered the supervision moves according to the possible functions of coaching supervision in the hope of making them easier to find should you look for a specific move in a given situation.

For the Restorative Function of Supervision

Coaching supervision has a restorative function when the supervision client feels burdened by their professional practice. It may be that they are saddened by an experience that one of their clients is facing or that they are overburdened and their work or something else is impacting their ability to function with joy and ease.

Coping Questions

The challenge with the restorative function of supervision is the balance between acknowledging the client's hardship and inviting focus on a way forward and awareness of resources and resilience. SF practice has often been accused of not taking the problems of clients seriously or being problem phobic. We do take clients' hardships seriously, acknowledging their suffering and difficulties. However, we do not want to analyse or invite focus on the suffering. We want to listen to the client's stories as much as clients need in order to feel heard and understood. Our experience is that if we do not do that and pivot to inquiring about desired outcomes or instances of resilience too quickly, the clients will try more intensively to convince us that their suffering is real, which is the opposite of what we want to invite.

Coping questions are a very good way of doing both: acknowledging the hardship and inviting a focus on resilience. In this move, the SF supervisor invites attention to how the client has been able to cope and what they have already done or experienced that is helpful. Here is a possible example:

Coaching supervision client: I would really like to talk about my experience in a recent coaching session. This was an initial session with an executive. She was not very open

	to coaching, and it seems like that the human resource department required her to take a few chemistry calls with coaches. In our meeting, she was really dismissive and downright rude to me. This hasn't left me and has kept me awake at night. How dare she treat me this way! I am hurt and I am angry and it is impacting my willingness to do new chemistry calls with executives. Can we talk about this?
Coaching supervisor:	I am so sorry to hear! I can see why this would impact you and I can feel your anger and frustration. I'm wondering how you have been able to cope since that meeting?
Coaching supervision client:	I have been distracting myself and then I tried to think about other things. Also, I have reminded myself of all the good chemistry calls that I have had.
Coaching supervisor:	Distracting yourself and reminding yourself of all the good chemistry calls that you've had. How has that been helpful?
Coaching supervision client:	It reminded me that I have so much more experience doing successful chemistry calls then the one experienced with this really rude client. I think it is important not to forget that.
Coaching supervisor:	Agreed!
Coaching supervision client:	Still, I would like to figure out why this meeting triggered me so much and what I can do to get back to my usual self-confidence.
Coaching supervisor:	You would like to figure out why this is triggering you and that you would like to get back to your usual self-confidence. Do you still want to share something about the chemistry meeting or are you happy for us to work on one or the other topic that you have mentioned?
Coaching supervision client:	I would like to tell you a little bit about what I think triggered me in this call and then I would like us to think about what I can do when and if this happens again.
Coaching supervisor:	How will you know that we have explored what triggered you enough so that we know when to move on?

As you can see in this example, there is a dance between the supervision client and supervisor around determining how much time needs to be spent on the "problem". In our view it is essential to partner with the client either verbally or nonverbally to determine when is a good time to move from acknowledging the hardship to crafting a way forward. When clients are in need of the restorative function of supervision, asking them how they've been able to cope broadens their view from a narrow focus on the problem or topic that is stressful for them to a more realistic and wider view of the situation. It is only natural that when clients are experiencing a hardship their thoughts are around that topic and they forget all the resources and resilience that they also have. The SF supervisor will invite attention to the broader picture.

Scaling

Scaling questions are also very useful in supervision sessions around the restorative function of coaching supervision. Here is the general structure of scaling questions:

"On the scale of zero to 10 where 10 is a good scenario and 0 is the opposite, where are you now?"

"What tells you that you are already at X?"

"What are you noticing that tells you that you're already at X?"

"What are other people noticing about you that tells them that you're already at X?"

"Suppose you were one step higher on that scale, what would you be noticing?"

"What would other people be noticing?"

"How would they respond?"

"How would you respond to their response?"

The idea behind scaling questions is to invite clients to explore the observable signs of differences. They come across as measuring something as they contain numbers. However, scaling in coaching supervision is not about measuring anything, but it is about helping clients become aware of the small differences which they might use for their growth.

Scaling questions are known to many coaches as part of their coaching move repertoire. This is why we don't want to go into great detail here but just provide a few thoughts on what the coaching supervisor might take care of when asking a scaling question.

Scaling Doesn't Have to Involve Numbers

As scaling questions are about identifying useful differences and not about measuring, it is not necessary to use numbers. In fact, the numbers in the scaling question are metaphors: they stand for situations. The supervisor can also use any kind of metaphor that the client is bringing, for example, climbing a mountain where success is when the peak has been reached. Other metaphors could be crossing a bridge or the colours of the sunset.

Describe 0 and 10 in Ways That Allow a Coaching Supervision Client to Pick a Number Somewhere in the Middle

In the restorative function of coaching supervision, the function of the scaling question is to allow supervision clients to identify strengths and resources. This is much easier if the question is phrased in a way that allows the client to pick a number somewhere in the middle rather than for example rating their situation at 0. If that happens the coaching supervisor can always go back to coping questions. However, framing 0 and 10 also has an influence. If the supervision client is very optimistic, the supervisor can use a more optimistic 10. Here are some examples:

"On a scale of zero to 10, where 10 is that you are starting to become a little bit optimistic that you can feel better about this client and zero is there is no chance at all, where are you now?"

"On a scale of zero to 10, where 10 is that you are confident that you can solve this situation with this client and 0 is the opposite, where are you now?"

"On a scale of zero to 10, where 10 is that you know that you will figure out what to do and 0 is the opposite, where are you now?"

Depending on the client's optimism the coach supervisor might choose any one of these scaling questions.

Viennese Basement Scale

What happens when the supervision client answers that they are at zero and have no hope? Here, the coaching supervisor might use a move called the "Viennese basement scale". It is said to have been invented by coaches working with the famously grumpy inhabitants of Vienna. If the client is not very hopeful, the supervisor might ask when it was worse. Now this sounds like not a very SF question, but hang on. As scaling is about identifying useful differences the supervisor might then go on by saying: "So now it is a little bit better than when it was at its worst? What makes it a little bit better?" This, again, is an invitation to describe useful differences.

Exceptions, Instances and Unique Outcomes

Another invitation of the supervisor may be to invite the client to describe a situation that was slightly better than usual. The wording for this move varies across social constructionist approaches. In the older literature on Solution Focus practices we find the word "exceptions". The more recent literature uses "instances" of the preferred future already happening and narrative practice talks about "unique outcomes". Each of these words carries a slightly different meaning. An "exception" presupposes that there is an enduring problem. "Unique outcomes" also presumes that generally the outcomes are less favourable, and "Instances" assumes that a preferred future is already happening at least partially, which in our view is the most useful way of looking at the situation.

Questions about instances invite the client to describe glimpses of the desired state already happening. Here are a few examples:

"You have described a lot of difficulties with this client and how you would like to be more self-confident. When did you see a little bit of that self-confidence showing up already?"

"What were you doing when it happened?"

"Who would be least surprised that you were able to show confidence in this situation?"

"What does this person know about you that would not have surprised them?"

Good Intentions of the Supervision Client

Assuming that supervision clients have good intentions with what they're doing is a very helpful attitude for any SF coaching supervisor. Of course, supervision clients sometimes mess up. They act in ways that are less than helpful for clients or they might even border on unethical behaviour.

In these cases it is necessary for the coaching supervisor to allow an exploration of what can be done better next time and invite reflection on the supervision client's behaviour. The supervisor could ask the client about their intentions and what they wanted to achieve and then explore other more professional or ethical ways of reaching the same goal. The alternative could be to explore the relationship the coaching supervision client would like to have with the intention they were holding. For example, a coach might have provided hands-on assistance to a client's project rather than coaching the client to do it themselves. An exploration might yield that the coach's intention was to be helpful. The supervisor and supervision client could then explore what it is about being helpful that is important to the supervision client and what would other ways of being helpful be that would be more in line with coaching.

For the Professional/Personal Development Function of Supervision

The professional/personal development function of supervision is best served by the supervisor when they are supporting the supervision client as a partner in the planning of their own learning. SF coaching sees the client as the expert for their own lives; SF coaching supervision assumes that supervision clients are best served if they are treated as the experts of their own learning. We want to support our supervision clients to become autonomous learners who are not only responsible for the content of their own learning and development but also supported in their discovery of which learning processes work best for them. In the following you will find the description of a few moves that may be helpful to do this.

Externalising and Reauthoring

Externalising and reauthoring are moves from narrative practice (White, 1995, 2007). They beautifully connect what the supervision client would like to develop or learn with the identity of the supervision client as a coach. The International Coaching Federation calls this distinction coaching "the what" and coaching "the who". In parallel, we could say that through externalising and reauthoring SF supervision invites the supervision of "the what" and "the who".

Let's say the supervision client wants to reflect on their discomfort coaching someone who is very different from themselves. A concrete example that I remember is a supervision client who was very uncomfortable coaching someone with a lot of tattoos and piercings. Here is how the externalising and reauthoring moves worked in this case:

Externalising

Coaching supervisor:	Do you have a name for your feeling of discomfort when you are in the presence of this client?
Coaching supervision client:	Yes, I call it "my inner bourgeois".
Coaching supervisor:	And what is your bourgeois keeping you from doing?
Coaching supervision client:	The bourgeois is keeping me from accepting people who are different than my norm. He tells me that I should stay away from people who are not like me, that I should be disgusted by everything that's not "prim and proper".
Coaching supervisor:	Sounds like you would like to accept people who are different, am I picking up what's important to you?
Coaching supervision client:	Yes of course. That is a big part of who I want to be as a coach. I want to be accepting of diversity and I want to be able to coach a wide array of people.
Coaching supervisor:	What kind of relationship would you like to have with the bourgeois?

Coaching supervision client: I would like to acknowledge that I do have a middle-class upbringing and that that shapes my perspective. I want to continue cherishing what this gave to me. So, I want to acknowledge and keep the bourgeois like a friend from high school; someone I remember fondly but not necessarily have any relationship with him at present.

Coaching supervisor: If you had that kind of relationship with your inner bourgeois, what difference would that make to the coaching with your pierced client?

Coaching supervision client: I think I would be more accepting and would feel less discomfort.

Coaching supervision: And how would your client notice?

You can see how externalising serves to create distance between the person of the client and the problem. The language moves from "my discomfort" to "my inner bourgeois" to "your bourgeois" to "the bourgeois", enlarging the distance. The question about the relationship the supervision client would like to have with their feelings helps to invite the client to consider options that were maybe not available before. Externalising and reauthoring are often connected. Here is an example how this may play out in a supervision session:

Coaching supervision client: My client would notice that I'm looking at him more. I wouldn't even be thinking about his piercings and tattoos and would just move on collaborating with him. I would be curious about him in a gentle and accepting way.

Coaching supervisor: Who would be least surprised if you told them that you'd managed to treat someone who is very different from you like that?

Coaching supervision client: Oh, I know my friend Jim from high school.

Coaching supervisor: What does Jim know about you that makes him not surprised?

Coaching supervision client: When I was in high school with Jim, he went through a phase of smoking pot and hanging out with a wild crowd. I didn't let that influence our friendship. I was simply able to accept it and kept Jim as my friend.

Coaching supervisor: What does that say about you as a person and as a coach?

Coaching supervision client: I think I am a very accepting person when I genuinely like someone. And I do like my clients a lot.

Coaching supervisor:	Would you like to think a bit about how you might act with your pierced client when you connect with your acceptance?
Coaching supervision client:	Yes of course. That's really what I would like!

In this example you can see how the conversation oscillates between talking a little bit more abstractly about who the supervision client is and wants to be and more concretely about the observable signs of what would happen. There are many moves that a supervisor may invite here. You might talk about the client as "the best coach they can be", or "how they would like to show up as a coach" or talk about whatever it is that the supervision client values highly about themselves personally or professionally.

Miracle Question

The miracle question is a move that is very famous in SF practice. It is almost a hallmark of the approach. What is important is that the miracle question, just as reauthoring or externalising is not just one question but a series of invitations. In contrast to externalising and reauthoring the miracle question does without a lot of abstraction. The client is invited to imagine their preferred future in observable detail. The coaching supervisor invites a rich description of the preferred future, how other people might respond and how the client might respond to their response and so on. An example might be:

Coaching supervisor:	Suppose we end this session and you go home and do whatever it is that you plan to do for the rest of the day. And at some time in the evening you get tired, you probably will go and brush your teeth, and you will go to bed. And as you're sleeping a miracle happens. And the miracle is that you have turned into the accepting coach that you would like to be. But as you are sleeping you cannot know that this miracle has happened.
What is the first sign the next morning that will tell you:	"Wow a miracle has happened"?
Coaching supervision client:	I would wake up and feel at ease looking forward to my day and also looking forward to meeting my client.
Coaching supervisor:	Who might notice that you are at ease?
Coaching supervision client:	My husband would notice.
Coaching supervisor:	What would he be noticing?
Coaching supervision client:	I would be smiling and maybe even singing a little song.
Coaching supervisor:	How would he respond?

Coaching supervision client:	He would be surprised but it would probably also put him in a good mood.
Coaching supervisor:	How would you respond to his good mood?
Coaching supervision client:	It would also strengthen my good mood and I would give him a big hug.
Coaching supervisor:	And how would he respond?

By inviting detailed descriptions of the desired future, the supervision client becomes more able to recognise when this preferred future happens. As the client is filling the images of their preferred future with images from their present or past experience, it also becomes more tangible and seems more likely to happen.

For the Quality Assurance and Ethical Guidance Function of Supervision

There are a few scenarios that call for the quality assurance and ethical guidance function of supervision: the supervision client may have a case that they are unsure of, the supervision client notices a potential ethical breach on their part, the supervision client may have a question about the quality of their coaching or the supervisor notices that the supervision client might have done something in a better way or even acted in a way that was not ethical. The main distinction is whether the supervisor or the supervision client is noticing a gap between the desired quality or ethical conduct and the actual quality and ethical conduct of the supervision client.

If the supervisor is noticing the ethical or quality gap, the supervisor needs to have the skills to mention this to the supervision client in such a way that it will not influence their relationship negatively. It is crucial that the supervisor continues to assume that the supervision client did not have any negative intentions or deliberately made a mistake.

In coaching, the coach might ask a coaching client for permission to share an observation as they may or may not be relevant to what the client wants to achieve. This is different in coaching supervision. It is a supervisor's responsibility to notice and mention to the supervision client when something might have negatively impacted the supervision client's client. The supervisor can recount what they heard the supervision client express about their conduct and check with the supervision client whether they have understood correctly. The supervisor can then ask for the supervision client's intentions and perspectives on the issue. A supervisor might bring in the relevant ethical frameworks and ask the supervision client to reflect.

As stated earlier, being SF does not mean being problem phobic. If a "mistake" happened, both coaching supervisor and supervision client can look at what happened, what the coach intended and ultimately how to act on this intention and better ways the next time. Supervisor and supervision client might also talk about how the supervision client may repair the situation if the client of the supervision client was negatively impacted by the supervision client's behaviour.

When to Give Advice

"Advice contains the word 'vice'" is a saying often used in the SF community, and in most instances, SF practitioners would stay clear of it as much as they can. As coaching supervision also has a quality assurance function, advice has a different position. This becomes apparent when you compare a coach's response to an error of their clients with a supervisor's response. The supervisor will partially be held responsible for the quality and ethical conduct of their supervision clients. After all, the clients of the supervision client feel assured that the supervision client is taking supervision and is investing in reflection and professional growth. Therefore advice plays a different role in coaching supervision.

We recommend to save any advice until after the supervision client has reflected themselves. In the metaphor of the gallery, the so-called gift shop is a good place. Supervisor and supervision client have agreed on a "ticket" which may have been initiated by the supervisor in the quality assurance function of supervision. The supervision client has reflected on their preferred future and on instances of the preferred future already happening. In the gift shop, the supervision client has come up with signs of improvement and maybe some possible experiments. Here it is quite easy for the supervisor to add to the supervision client's ideas if the supervision clients would like to hear them or if the supervision client's solutions can be added to by the supervisor. Sometimes there simply might be things that the supervision client does not know and that are important for the supervision client to learn.

Supervision With the Client Present

As mentioned previously, the SF approach focuses on interactions and relationships. Taking this stance, it is actually quite strange that supervision usually happens with only one person of the relevant systems and the coaching relationships present. In SF therapy, there is a long tradition of case consultations with clients and therapists. Insoo Kim Berg and Steve de Shazer often saw therapists and their clients together with the aim of strengthening their relationship. We think that this modality is not used often enough and has a lot of potential to help coaches and their clients to have even more fruitful discussions. In the following you will find some structures and moves that may be helpful should you decide to venture out and see a supervision client and their client together.

Strengthening the Collaboration

The aim of doing supervision with the supervision client and their client is to strengthen the collaboration between them. Rather than walking through a whole gallery with the supervision client and their client the supervisor can start the session by asking both parties what they are appreciating in their collaboration. As always, it is important to invite concrete descriptions: "When we were talking about the preparation of my presentation, I really appreciate how we went through the presentation in great detail", rather than: "I like that you're thorough". As a simple next step the supervisor might use the scaling move: "On a scale of zero to 10, where 10 is you are the best coach and client pair thinkable and zero is the opposite where are you?", "How would you notice that you are even one step higher on that scale?", "What is the coach doing and what is the client doing?".

The supervisor will stress that both client and supervision client are responsible for their relationship. Both can do things to make it more fruitful and both have done things to make it fruitful.

Outsider Witness Structures

Outsider witness moves come from narrative practice. They are a really interesting and strengthening way to leverage the situation when you have supervision clients and their clients together in a room.

The supervisor first explains the process and asks whether both supervision client and their client are happy to engage with it. In the following we will use the word "coach" for the supervision client and the word "client" for the supervision client's client in the hope that this is less confusing. The structure then is as follows:

- Both coach and client describe someone that they know who listens really well. The supervisor asks them to listen to each other with the ears of that person. The supervisor also explains that after each contribution the other will retell what stood out for them in what they just heard. The supervisor asks both parties to mentally note what seems important to the other including important phrases and words that they mention.
- The client starts by describing their experience of the coaching process and relationship. This can include all the good experiences, the not so good experiences and the experiences that that coach's client would rather not have had.
- Meanwhile the coach listens with the open ears of the person who can listen very well and takes the mental note of all the things that seem important to the client.
- The supervisor then asks the coach to retell what they have heard.
- Then the supervisor asks the coach to share what resonates with the coach and what the client has said and mention which ripple effects this will have in their life.
- Then coach and client switch roles and the coach now shares their experience of the coaching relationship and the client listens with open ears, retells, shares resonances and ripple effects.

Usually this is a very touching process and strengthens the relationship between coach and client as well as helping both identify what they are doing that is helping the client and the coach to grow.

Common Topics in Individual Supervision

There are various topics that emerge when doing individual coaching supervision, and we offer some common topics shared by the authors, mentioned in other chapters and shared by other coaching supervisors. For a comprehensive review, refer to Chapter 14 on Common Topics that offers suggestions and questions for the supervisor to engage the learning of the supervision client. Individual supervision topics are organised under four functions of supervision below.

Restorative Function

- Coach is experiencing burnout.
- Coach is feeling burdened by their professional practice.
- Coach is upset about a coaching session.

Professional Growth/Personal Development

- Coach wants to build their confidence in coaching senior executives.
- Coach seeks feedback on a coaching session to improve their skills.
- Coach wants to process areas he feels he needs to develop.

Quality Assurance and Ethical Functions

- Coach is uncertain about boundaries and potential conflict of interest.
- Coach is uncertain as to how to manage increasing demands from stakeholders.
- Coach wants to process biases that are getting in the way of their coaching.

Managerial and Commercial – Business Development

- Coach wants to discuss business development for his new venture.
- Coach is interested in latest market research and best practice in youth coaching.
- Coach wants to explore how to build a successful coaching practice.

Conclusion

We have included several different processes that a supervisor can use to engage the learning of their supervision client. Whether using "moves" or the "gallery" metaphor, both offer a rich resource in which to experiment and develop your SF supervision style.

Reflective Exercise

- Reflect and consider which of the ideas in the chapter resonate with you.
- Which of the SF moves would you like to try out?

References

McKergow, M. (2021). *The next generation of solution focused practice. Stretching the world for new opportunities and progress.* Routledge.

White, M. (1995). *Re-authoring lives. Interviews & essays.* Dulwich Centre Publications.

White, M. (2007). *Maps of narrative practice.* W. W. Norton.

5 Demonstrating Ethical Coaching Supervision Practice

Svea van der Hoorn

Introduction

Ethics is central to professional practice, but is often engaged with from a rarefied rather than grounded perspective. Many coaches regard ethics as a necessary, but dry and somewhat boring compliance requirement. This chapter breathes life into how coaching supervision can support coaches to live ethical coaching practice. The International Coaching Federation (ICF) Codes of Ethics and Core Competencies as well as the European Mentoring and Coaching Council (EMCC) Global Code of ethics and competences are brought to life as talk to be walked, not only talked. The Solution Focused resource activation stance to exploring ethical dilemmas encourages data-based decision-making, while not losing sight of the fact that coaching happens in the fluidity of conversations and relationships. Scenarios are offered in which the reader can experiment with a framework for ethical decision-making. The issue of unintended unethical conduct is considered in relation to bounded ethicality and ethical fading.

The chapter includes ethical issues arising in relation to coaching and coaching supervision practice with mandated clients, working with multiple stakeholders, and managing dual relationships with clients, for example, when working as an internal coach. The ethics around referral are reflected upon in the light of learnings from the disruptions.

Welcome to the World of Ethics

Ethics are the principles that guide our behaviour towards making decisions/ choices that contribute to the common good of all. These principles provide necessary guidance to ensure equity and fair discrimination. To discriminate is something that is part of everyday life, for example, when clients select a coach from a pool of coaches. Coaches do this when they make decisions about fees they charge and availability. Coaching is unregulated in most countries which raises questions about risk of harm. Ethics are what guides us to tell the truth, for example, about qualifications, training, scope of practice, to keep our promises and to act with compassion. However, demonstrating ethical coaching practice and ethical coaching supervision practice is neither easy nor straightforward,

DOI: 10.4324/9781003390527-5

given that ethics are aspirational. They guide but do not dictate the conduct of coaches and coaching supervisors. Translating the principles into practices that are contextually appropriate and aligned to clients' best interests involves discernment, self-awareness, managing bias and blindspots, and the courage to engage in conversations with a view to resolve dilemmas rather than fuel conflict.

Concerns about potential ethical dilemmas are commonly encountered by coaching supervisors. These can arise from the coaching supervision client and/or from the coaching supervisor. Engaging with managing or resolving these ethical dilemmas is one of the activities that sets coaching supervision apart from coaching. It highlights the paradox of the coaching supervisor needing to be both a steward for coaching ethics, as well as a supporter of coaches as they develop ethical maturity and their self-regulation capacity. This paradox demands of coaching supervisors to develop skills to address ethical issues in coaching supervision, rather than to remain silent, to be able to promote ethical maturity by engaging with the coaching supervision client's ethical decision-making framework and being able to move between the abstract/world of ideas and the applied/world of actions, with both rigour and compassion. What may seem a daunting set of demands becomes manageable for Solution Focused coaching supervisors who adopt a resource-oriented stance as their starting point. We invite you to consider the following questions to check what you already have in your ethical coaching practice and what you might like to learn, add, refine or update:

- What are the values and Code/s of Ethics of any professional coaching organisations you align with and/or are a member of? How well do these align with your personal values?
- How accessible is information on ethical coaching practice to you? Is it quick and easy to access like your coffee/tea cup, your supply of tea and coffee, and anything else you rely on daily? Or tucked away in a filing cabinet, a folder on your computer that you've forgotten about, or somewhere in the notes from your coach education?
- Where, and in what format would you like the information to be so that it is part of your work with coaching supervision clients as seamlessly as reaching out for what you need in order to make a cup of tea/coffee?
- All Codes of Ethics propose the duty of "do good, not harm". What do you require of yourself in your everyday life and work moments that guides you to stay aligned with duty?
- Who are your go-to people when you are concerned about ethical practice? As coaching supervisors we encourage all our coaching supervision clients to have at least three ethics buddies they can contact at any time of the day or night for a quick (15 minutes) touch base, to clarify, confirm, contain and then decide about how to proceed. This may take longer than 15 minutes and often does, but the clarify, confirm and contain aspects can be done in a 15-minute disciplined reflective practice style conversation. This is usually sufficient to cope and to prevent things from getting worse for long enough to then do the more expanded reflective practice that the dilemma may require.

Confusions and Misunderstandings About Ethics

Before moving into exploring ethical coaching supervision practice, we pause to consider some confusions and common misunderstandings about ethics and ethical coaching practice.

- Ethics is interconnected with but not synonymous with the law. Turning to the law or using legal language and argument building is often a natural first step, but can even be counterproductive when responding to an ethical dilemma. While most Codes of Ethics will include that coaches and coaching supervisors are expected to abide by relevant laws and local customs, this alone is insufficient. Hence coaching organisations like ICF and EMCC provide values as guidelines as well as Codes of Ethics that speak to what coaches and coaching supervisors should take into consideration when making decisions and to self-regulate their conduct.

- Ethics is interconnected with but not synonymous with morality. A similar error is made when the law is found to be insufficient to resolve an ethical dilemma, and morality is turned to for guidance. "A person is moral if they conform to the established practices and customs of the group in which they are. A person is ethical if they voluntarily obligate themselves to live in the light of an ideal good. The two notions are distinct but not necessarily incompatible … as is evident in the character of even the most decadent society" (Weiss, 1942, p. 381).

- Ethics is less about right and wrong, and more about making decisions and taking action in the face of uncertainty, ambiguity, volatility and diversity. Ethical fading is commonly encountered by coaching supervisors when listening to accounts of why coaches decided to act as they did. Ethical fading occurs when the ethical guidelines fade from view, often being eclipsed by over-focusing on another aspect informing a decision, such as profitability, reputation or not wanting to create discomfort. The coach convinces themselves, and sometimes the coaching supervisor, of the rightness of their focus and logic, leading to the ethical aspects of the decision being dismissed or minimised. Which may well lead to an ethical complaint being lodged when other parties do take into consideration the ethical guidelines relevant to the decision (McCombs School of Business, n.d.).

- Ethics is objective and neutral; ethics is universal and transcends diversity and context. The rise of online working during the COVID pandemic has led to coaching supervisors to become increasingly exposed to the wide variety of local customs and laws, norms and values, and ways of practising coaching that exist. This has led to questioning the idea that coaching supervisors can be objective or neutral and what to be instead? Declaration of bias and blindspots and the willingness to explore these has become one way to manage the diversity and complexity in a transparent and collaborative manner.

Ethical Coaching Supervision Practice

The worlds of ethical coaching practice and coaching supervision are expansive when it comes to information – whether research-based, grounded in theory, or placed in the public domain via popular literature and social media posts. We propose the following as sufficient stepping stones for coaching supervisors to equip themselves with in order to navigate the turbulent waters arising from ethical dilemmas. They also assist with freeing coaching supervision clients from being stuck in the doldrums of outdated information, making ethical decisions that are context oblivious or insufficiently aware, and the swirling vortexes of bias and blindspots.

Given that ethical dilemmas are by their nature ambiguous and require engagement with uncertainty, tension and contradictions, we offer some frames of reference that can provide coaching supervisors and their coaching supervision clients with a sense of exploring within sufficient containment.

Definitions of Coaching

Every definition of coaching will give direction in terms of what the purpose, focus and benefits are that the coach is promising and hence is ethically bound to deliver. For example, the ICF definition describes the relationship between coach and client as one of "partnering in a thought-provoking and creative process that inspires the client to maximise their personal and professional potential" (International Coaching Federation, n.d.). The emphasis is on a relationship characterised by partnering and a process that inspires learning and growth. Then there are definitions of coaching that arise from theories and models. Some coach education is model specific, some familiarise students to multiple models, some are eclectic and some do not include explicit focus on theories and models. A discussion about definitions can be a useful starting point for coaching supervisors and their coaching supervision clients to check the alignment and discordance between the definitions of coaching that they each are guided by. How to manage these similarities and differences can be built into the coaching supervision agreement.

From the coaching supervisor's point of view, it is important to check whether the coach is a member of or holds certification from a coaching organisation. There is an expectation that this binds coaches to practise within the definitions or make themselves vulnerable to a complaint. It is not recommended nor required that coaching supervisors know all the definitions of coaching. Rather, talking about the definitions offers an opportunity to check, reflect and clarify. Questions that can be useful include:

- Where can we read about the definition/s of coaching that guide your practice?
- Which aspects of the definition are you at ease with expressing in your practice?

- Which aspects do you tend to ignore, minimise or over-amplify?
- How do you self-regulate and quality control to ensure you are delivering what the buyers of your coaching expect from you, given your membership/certification/qualifications?
- How would you like us to take into consideration your definition of coaching and/or adherence to a specific coaching model/theory as part of our coaching supervision work that is relevant to you maintaining professional standards?

Ethical Coaching Practice as Defined by Coaching Organisations

In addition to definitions of coaching, the coaching organisations offer guidelines to their members in terms of values, a Code of Ethics and standards of practice. For example, EMCC Competence 4 binds members to "promotes professional standards – professional behaviour and conduct when working with clients/supervisees that is committed to delivering the level of service that may reasonably be expected of a practising member" (EMCC Global, 2015).

Codes of Ethics are often consulted outside of rather than during coaching sessions by coaches. However, Codes of Ethics are often a regular part of coaching supervision. When entering into a coaching supervision contract which involves meeting regularly, for example, monthly or quarterly, the following questions can be explored with the coaching supervision client:

- What does ethical coaching practice look like in relation to the Codes of Ethics that your coaching practice is aligned to/governed by?
- What are your personal and professional values as a coach?
- What kind of ethical coaching practice do you want to be known for?

In the same way that coaches are required/advised to align their coaching practice with the ethical conduct espoused in Codes of Ethics, so coaching supervisors too are required/advised that their coaching supervision should be aligned to coaching supervision standards of practice and ethical guidelines. These are available from coaching supervision accreditation agencies, for example, EMCC offers a framework for coaching supervision which is research and feedback based (EMCC Global, 2019). EMCC proposes the following eight core competences, clustered into four categories, as what coaching supervisors can and should use to self-regulate their coaching supervision practice:

A **Contracting**

1 Manages the supervision contract and process

B **The Functions of Supervision**

2 Facilitates development
3 Provides support
4 Promotes professional standards

C The Capacity of the Supervisor

5 Self-awareness
6 Relationship awareness
7 Systemic awareness

D Working with Groups

8 Facilitates group supervision

These EMCC coaching supervision competences are linked to 40 behavioural indicators, which provide coaching supervisors with more detailed awareness of what offering quality coaching supervision involves.

The EMCC Global Code of Ethics was established in 2016, with the most recent revision being undertaken in 2021 (https://www.emccglobal.org/leadership-development/ethics/). It proposes four categories, namely:

- Terminology
- Working with clients
- Professional conduct
- Excellent practice

In 2024, the ICF had not yet introduced core competencies for coaching supervisors. However, the titles of the sections of the 2019 Code of Ethics in themselves provide coaching supervisors with guidance and direction about their role in supporting coaches to align their practice with the ICF Code of Ethics (https://coachingfederation.org/ethics/code-of-ethics), namely:

- Section I: Responsibilities to clients
- Section II: Responsibilities to practice and performance
- Section III: Responsibility to professionalism
- Section IV: Responsibility to society

Navigating Ethical Dilemmas in Coaching Supervision

Coaching supervisors are often the go to people when coaches are concerned about potential ethical dilemmas in their coaching practice. However, not every concern or dilemma is an ethical dilemma as defined by the Codes of Ethics. Before considering how to navigate an ethical dilemma with a coaching supervision client, we invite you to pause and reflect on the following:

- If you are already offering coaching supervision – what are the most common ethical dilemmas you have faced as a coaching supervisor?
- If not yet offering coaching supervision, what ethical issues have you faced as a coach that you would look to a coaching supervisor for support with?

Applying an Ethical Decision-Making Framework

Every ethical dilemma brings with it choices, decisions and actions. We offer the following way to structure conversation, informed by and adapted from Passmore (2009):

- What bias and/or blindspots are evoked when you first read the scenario? How can you take care not to skew your decision-making towards confirming or avoiding or ignoring these?
- Which category/ies of the ICF Code and section/s of the EMCC Global Code is/are relevant to the dilemma?
- Which specific ICF and/or EMCC Code of Ethics standard/s are relevant to the dilemma (there may be more than one)? This requires the coaching supervision client and coaching supervisor to engage in narrowing the dilemma to which particular category/ies it is relevant to, and then continuing to select the particular ethical standard/s that need to be considered in resolving the dilemma.
- Solution Focused coaching supervisors then invite the coaching supervision client to reflect on what strengths and resources can be drawn on. These are thought of broadly, including the stakeholders, the context and society, rather than being limited to only the coach and their coaching client.
- What bias/blindspots may be relevant to this dilemma? This question invites being transparent and aware, rather than attempting to hold a position of objectivity and neutrality.
- What guidance is offered by the ICF insights and considerations for ethics (ICE) statements and the EMCC Global Code that can be drawn on when working to resolve this dilemma?
- What timelines need to be considered in resolving this dilemma? Some pragmatic questions posed by Solution Focused coaching supervisors include "By when do you need to be seen to be responding to this dilemma?" "What is the smallest signal that you need to communicate that will tell people you are responding to this dilemma?" "By when will this dilemma no longer be a dilemma that you have choice about?" It may evaporate, be replaced by a further dilemma, become an official complaint, jump to a different context, for example, legal proceedings or social media public domain posting.
- Who are the relevant stakeholders to be included in resolving this dilemma? It may seem strange that stakeholder inclusion appears only here in the sequence. However, premature decisions about who to include can lead to outliers not being considered for inclusion and/or the role of more obvious stakeholders being over-emphasised.
- And, who and what else should we take into account/consider? This is a very powerful question that coaching supervisors carry the accountability for asking especially when the coaching supervision client may be keen to move to decision and action as the stress of the dilemma decreases.

We now offer a few ethical dilemmas that illustrate what coaching supervision clients may bring to coaching supervision. We invite you to slip into the coaching supervisor seat and experiment with applying the above framework to each scenario.

Scenario A

The coaching supervision client says that a professional acquaintance has just referred a colleague to them for coaching. This person is very enthusiastic about beginning the coaching straight away, based on the flattering introduction. The coaching supervision client is aware that the person does not have a clear idea of what coaching really is, nor what the coaching client's responsibilities are. The referred person is urging the coaching supervision client to not worry about preparing a coaching contract before the coaching starts. They are keen to have a session as soon as possible and happy to deal with the contract in the next few weeks. The coaching supervision client is very keen to secure this coaching assignment as it will be reputation enhancing and also has a significant fee attached to it due to the glowing referral. The coaching supervision client requested an urgent coaching supervision appointment as the clock is ticking and they saw just before they arrived that the prospective coaching client had gone ahead and booked an appointment in their digital calendar. The link to their calendar is included in their e-mail signature.

Scenario B

The coaching supervision client works for 50% of their time as an internal coach, and for the remainder of the time in the on-site health clinic as an occupational health and safety nurse. The topic they bring to coaching supervision is what to do when in a coaching session an employee discloses they are considering harm to self or others. The coaching supervision client describes that this is happening more frequently and thinks that it has to do with people feeling more comfortable to reveal this in coaching, which they understand is more confidential than what they may say when visiting the health clinic. The coaching supervision client says that there is an expectation that emotions such as shame, anger, frustration and even revenge can be discussed in coaching, but that the health clinic is a place where medication, diet and exercise and/or referrals to specialist services are the likely outcome. The coaching supervision client mentions that what is stressful for them is that they report to two different managers, who do not get along. The health clinic manager thinks coaching is a lot of talk that gets no results. The coaching manager thinks the health clinic manager is too attached to a medical model way of dealing with any and all emotional difficulties employees may experience. Both these managers have recently started reporting to a new line manager, who has made known that coaching needs to know its scope of practice, and stay within its scope.

Scenario C

The coaching supervision client says that they and their coaching client are becoming frustrated at the lack of progress the coaching client is making, both during and between the coaching sessions. There have been three sessions so far of the contracted six-session package. The coaching supervision client thinks the coaching client would be better served by counselling/therapy as the coaching client refers repeatedly to past experiences and current emotions which get in the way of them putting changes discussed in the coaching sessions into action between sessions. They say they meant to, but could not. At the end of the last session the coaching client expressed that perhaps focusing more on their feelings and how to manage them is what will let them make progress. After the session the coaching client sent the coach an email asking whether the coach's approach to coaching allows for a more emotional focus? They are experiencing the coaching as very focused on them changing their behaviours, whereas the coaching they did with a previous coach allowed for much more managing of their emotions. The coaching supervision client does not disagree that perhaps the coaching client would prefer a more emotion-focused approach. However, they think they would be failing in their duty to the coaching client if they did not raise a referral to counselling/therapy rather than to another style of coaching. They are concerned about the coaching client's descriptions of how they are "losing it" at work and with family members. The coaching client has not given details of what "losing it" involves. The coaching supervision client has said to the coaching supervisor "this is a seriously intense personality who does not hold back with their words. I am not sure how ugly things could become if they were challenged or not given what they think they are entitled to".

Now that you have explored the scenarios using the decision-making framework, gather your learnings via these reflection questions:

- What did you notice from engaging with, and then managing your bias/blindspot responses to each scenario?
- Which parts of the decision-making framework did you find clear and simple to implement? What does this tell you about your strengths in ethical decision-making?
- Which parts of the decision-making framework were more demanding? How might you become more fit at these?

Based on your learnings and your reflections, what activities, conversations and perusal of resources would support you in developing your ability to be a coaching supervisor who is well equipped to do a good job at supporting coaching supervision clients who face an ethical dilemma in their coaching practice?

Ethical Fading: It Is Not Done Until It Is Done

Whilst ethical decision-making stretches us, what is even more demanding is the taking of action in relation to what emerges from the ethical decision-making process. A common error in coaching supervision is to think deciding on ethical conduct is complete once the confusion, tensions and contradictions that arise from the dilemma are eased or even resolved at the level of thinking. The coaching supervision client no longer feels perplexed or stuck or confused. The process appears complete when this thought appears "Now I know what to do!" In fact, this is a moment of vulnerability where coaching supervisors need to support the coaching supervision client to face "And how committed am I to implementing the actions that flow from my decision making?"

Bounded ethicality and ethical fading help us understand why using an ethical decision-making framework and committing to following through with the actions that flow from this process are so necessary and something that coaching supervisors can play a significant role in supporting. Rees et al. (2019) offer the following insights into how unintended unethical behaviour arises. Bounded ethicality occurs where people engage in "behaviour that is contradictory to their values without realising that they are doing so. We further argue that ethical fading – when individuals do not see the ethical implications of the situation or their action – is central to explaining why this occurs" (Rees et al., 2019, p. 27). A verbal clue that signals that a coaching supervision exploration of bounded ethicality and/or ethical fading may be wise is when coaching supervisors hear "but that wasn't my intention" or find themselves listening to explanations and justifications about why other factors were/are more important in guiding actions than ethical considerations. The purposeful application of a decision-making framework such as the one offered above makes the likelihood of stepping into bounded ethicality and/or ethical fading less likely.

Setting Up Ethical Coaching Supervision

After the deep dive into some of what coaching supervisors need to be prepared for in their work, this chapter now moves to how coaching supervisors might go about setting up their coaching supervision practice in an ethically alive and aligned way. We place this here in the chapter deliberately. Without first exploring what coaching supervisors may be faced with in their coaching supervision practices, it is easy to fall into the trap of adopting a compliance-based approach, rather than an intentional and practice-informed approach.

Contracting: How We Start Can Make All the Difference

Twenty twenty hindsight is illuminating when it comes to identifying when was the earliest moment that a coaching supervision client could have detected clues that they needed to pay attention to the ethical implications of what was happening between them and their coaching client/s. Reflective practice often identifies the initial communication and the contracting phase as where many of the ethical dilemmas experienced by coaching supervision clients could have been prevented or where the foundation for collaborative resolution rather than conflict could have been put in place. Let us consider what contracting offers us in relation to not just relationship building but also to cultivating a space for ethical coaching conduct and practice. First, a few reflection questions:

If you are already offering coaching supervision

- What do you need to cover when setting up a new coaching supervision contract?
- What would the differences be if you were contracting with an individual coaching supervision client directly versus where you are employed by a third party to provide coaching supervision?
- What are the benefits and strengths of the coaching supervision you can offer coaching supervision clients? What are some of the limits/boundaries or your coaching supervision services? What coaching supervision requests are outside of what you offer?

If you are not yet offering coaching supervision/wish to look from the perspective of the coaching supervision client:

- Write a list of what information you would expect a coaching supervisor to make available to you so that you can decide on whether to enter into a coaching supervision contract with them.
- How would you describe the benefits you are looking for from coaching supervision?
- What criteria would you use to evaluate the fit between the benefits you are looking for and what the coaching supervisor offers? What clues would give you confidence that you are likely to benefit from the coaching supervision offered by a specific coaching supervisor?

Some Solution Focused questions for setting up supervision, with an individual include:

- What is the purpose of our coaching supervision?
- How can we tell that the time is being well used?
- How would you know this is value creating coaching supervision?
- How would your clients be able to tell you were undertaking coaching supervision that benefits them?
- How would colleagues/your manager be able to tell your coaching supervision was value-adding?

Some Solution Focused questions for setting up supervision, with a third party/buyer

- What does X want from the coaching supervision that you will be funding?
- What needs to happen for you to have confidence that this coaching supervision is money and time well spent?
- How will we all monitor that the coaching supervision is value-adding?
- Who is responsible for what record-keeping and information sharing?

Solution Focused coaching supervision encourages us to consider pre-session change as we start with a coaching supervision engagement. Rather than assuming the coaching supervision client is uninformed about coaching supervision, attention is paid to what the coaching supervision client's good reasons are for seeking coaching supervision and what they have already been doing to support themselves in ensuring that their coaching practice is guided by and meets ethical standards. Attention is also paid to descriptions of past success experiences by inviting them to describe benefits of previous coaching supervision they may have experienced, as well as how the coaching supervision made a difference to them and their practice.

Solution Focused coaching supervision views detail as essential to partnering/co-creation. Hence the contracting detail is seen not merely as practical, but rather as illuminating the interactional landscape within which the coaching supervisor and coaching supervision client will collaborate. Some practicalities to consider, discuss and explicitly agree on include venue, dates and times, frequency, duration, managing rescheduling and cancellation, payment, paperwork, contact details, emergency contact details, availability outside coaching supervision appointments and other support people and resources the coaching supervision client makes use of. An essential element in an ethically aligned coaching supervision contract is around the shared responsibility for the confidentiality afforded to the clients of the coaching supervision client. It is the coaching supervisor's accountability to make explicit that the coaching supervision client is responsible for obtaining permission to discuss their coaching work with the coaching supervisor. The benefits of establishing and maintaining a sufficiently detailed and fully explored contract include:

- encouraging collaboration, transparency, openness and rigour,
- clarifying roles, boundaries and responsibilities,
- formalising coaching supervision and accountability for ethical coaching practice,
- clarifying what resources will be drawn on and how ethical issues will be navigated if these arise and
- providing a document to refer back to if queries/issues.

Ultimately what coaching supervisors are seeking to offer is a safe space that is learning and growth promoting. Factors that will enhance or detract from this include what the coaching supervisor brings (experience, expertise, working style) what the coaching supervision client brings (experience, learning needs) and the interplay and navigation of the best hopes/expectations of both the coaching supervision client and the coaching supervisor. Thomas (2013) offers some positions to consider in relation to how a coaching supervisor shows up in the coaching supervision relationship and the dominant communication style associated with each. As you read these, which is the position and communication style that appeals to you most? When might you make use of the others, if ever? What are the implications of these reflections for what you offer coaching supervision clients? How will you communicate this to prospective clients so as to offer them the opportunity to make an informed decision about whether you are the coaching supervisor they would like to enter into a contractual working relationship with?

- Gatekeeper position: here the coaching supervisor is a steward of quality. This includes arbitrating over whether coaching supervision clients may belong to a community of practitioners, receive a qualification, or be licensed to offer a specific model/approach of coaching practice. Communication style: two by four – a prescriptive, norm-based coaching supervision, where the coaching supervisor requires specific actions from the coaching supervision client. What is required is clear and sufficiently detailed to be able to be externally evaluated. However, this style brings with it less responsibility for the coaching supervision client to be self-regulating and alignment seeking, rather than compliance oriented.
- Guru position: imparts expert knowledge on coaching practice which coaching supervision clients then seek to copy. Communication style: uses a semaphore type signalling system – "please pay attention to what I am saying". This is less direct than instructions that must be implemented, thus encouraging some critical thinking, reflective practice and self-reliance, but can be open to misunderstandings and hence evokes hesitancy and/or seeking external validation on the part of the coaching supervision client.
- Guide: collaborates with the coaching supervision client to foster learning which will elicit the coaching supervision client's own unique version of coaching practice. Communication style: metaphor-like relating of stories that create space for interpretation and choice by the coaching supervision client. This is a more indirect style which provides space for individual interpretation and decision, but also may not provide sufficient containment.

Some Specific Ethical Dilemmas That Coaching Supervision Contracting Can Minimise and/or Resolve

- Referral to other services: historically there has been a focus on the scope of coaching versus the scope of counselling/therapy. However, with the lockdowns and physical isolating required during the COVID pandemic in the 2020s, many coaches were faced with coaching clients bringing to their coaching issues which might under usual circumstances be deemed more suitable for referral to other services/professionals. For many coaching clients, the intensity of upheaval of their working and personal lives made them keen to maintain the trust and safety they experienced in their coaching, and not keen to be referred elsewhere, even if there was an accessible service. There was a rise in requests for support about how to manage remote working and the intrusion of work into home life, managing stress and strain due to fears of becoming physically ill, disruption to business and income generation, anxiety about how to fulfil responsibilities to employees and contractors, concerns about parenting children in times of global crises and a sense of a doomed future, and more. This wave of change and disruption brought into question the ethics of referral, especially under conditions where many of the usual referral resources were not operating, or operating with significant restrictions to accessibility. Solution Focused coaching supervision encouraged to keep things simple and pragmatic without crossing ethical boundaries. Questions like "What support CAN you offer your coaching client that will allow them to do the best they can with what IS available to them under current conditions, and without you ignoring or violating the ethical codes and standards you uphold?"

- Multiple stakeholders: the coaching supervisor may wish to draw on a concept from design thinking, namely, stakeholder mapping (https://www.interaction-design.org/literature/article/map-the-stakeholders). Having all stakeholders and the authority and interests mapped onto one page allows both the coaching supervisor and the coaching supervision client to engage with the complexities and potential ethical concerns and conflicts, without becoming caught in overwhelm.
- Mandated clients: coaching supervisors may find themselves working with non-voluntary coaching supervision clients and/or coaching supervision clients whose willingness to engage with coaching supervision is compliance-driven rather than by the desire for learning and growth. This is becoming more prevalent with the rise of coaching agents, for example coaching platforms where the business contract is forged not by the coaching supervision client themselves. Detailed contracting around roles and responsibilities, as well as around monitoring and evaluation of services is crucial. Equally important is the explicit identification of how concerns will be managed in terms of which ethical codes and standards of practice will be consulted about any ethical dilemmas. It is recommended by both the EMCC and ICF Codes of Ethics that there be explicit attention paid to how perception of conflicts of interests will be managed.
- Dual roles: similarly to the perception of conflicts of interests, the management of dual roles is considered crucial to ethical coaching supervision. This may arise from the coaching supervisor fulfilling more than one role,

for example, as a colleague and fellow employee with internal coaches, and as head of the coaching pool carrying the additional responsibility for quality assurance of the coaching offered in the organisation by offering coaching supervision to those in the coaching pool. Some of this dilemma can be resolved by sharing dilemmas and decisions with a coaching supervisor.

Next Steps

This concluding paragraph is intentionally not called "In conclusion". Demonstrating ethical coaching supervision is not an activity that has a conclusion. Rather it is an ever present accountability requiring attention, care and reflection by the coaching supervisor. With this in mind, we close the chapter with some reflection questions:

- What is our preferred way of maintaining an openness to learning and growth as regards ethical practice? Is this by reading, through conversations with peers, by attending formal education, by participating in conferences, summits, webinars and events?
- If you follow the EMCC guideline on regularity of an activity being key to maintaining quality and ethical alignment – one hour of supervision for every 35 hours of coaching and at least once a quarter, what is your timeline/rhythm for engaging in expanding and refreshing your coaching supervision expertise?
- Who are your go-to people that can help you stay clear about your ethical coaching supervision being and doing? These people should include at least one person who thinks very differently from you and is willing to engage you in contradictory debates, one person who has your back no matter how foolish they may think your conduct, and one person who stays steady when the perturbation of a potential ethical dilemma presents itself, often at an inopportune time.

References

EMCC Global. (2015). *EMCC competence framework*. https://www.emccglobal.org/wp-content/uploads/2018/10/EMCC-competences-framework-v2-EN.pdf

EMCC Global. (2019). *Supervision competence framework*. Retrieved from https://www.emccglobal.org/leadership-development/supervision/competences/

International Coaching Federation. (n.d.). *What is coaching?* Retrieved February 7, 2024, from https://coachingfederation.org/about

McCombs School of Business (n.d.). *Ethics unwrapped: Ethical fading*. Retrieved February 27, 2024, from https://ethicsunwrapped.utexas.edu/glossary/ethical-fading

Passmore, J. (2009). Coaching ethics: Making ethical decisions: Experts and novices. *The Coaching Psychologist, 5(1)*, 6–10.

Rees, M.R., Tenbrunsel, A.E., & Bazerman, M.H. (2019). Bounded ethicality and ethical fading in negotiations: Understanding unintended unethical behaviour. *Academy of Management Perspectives*, *33*(1), 26–42. https://doi.org/10.5465/amp.2017.0055

Thomas, F.N. (2013). *Solution-focused supervision*. Springer.

Weiss, P. (1942). Morality and ethics. *The Journal of Philosophy*, *39*(14), 381–385. https://doi.org/10.2307/2018625; https://www.jstor.org/stable/2018625

6   Case Supervision

Debbie Hogan, Jane Tuomola
and Sukanya Wignaraja

Introduction

Case supervision has a more specific focus than individual coaching supervision in that it focuses on the exploration of a specific client case, to enhance the quality of service to that particular client.

The tenets of the Solution Focused (SF) approach are described in detail in Chapter 3 (see pp. 27–42). This chapter describes how the SF tenets of pragmatism, curiosity, taking an interactional view, seeing progress and resources rather than deficits, apply when doing case supervision.

Common topics that typically arise in case supervision include:

- challenges related to establishing rapport,
- establishing clear coaching agreements related to goals and expectations,
- measuring progress or addressing obstacles related to goal achievement,
- enhancing client engagement,
- navigating cultural differences,
- handling difficult emotions,
- exploring reactions or possible biases that emerge,
- seeking guidance for personal growth,
- seeking feedback on coaching techniques and approaches and
- asking for advice.

In addition to describing a case, a coaching supervision client can also bring a recording of the session to listen together with the coaching supervisor. The differences between case supervision with a recording and International Coach Federation (ICF) mentor coaching are discussed.

The chapter offers an annotated transcript of an SF case supervision session which shows how an SF coaching supervisor approaches issues such as, how to offer advice, how to keep the focus on the interaction between the coaching supervision client and their client and how to move between the different functions of supervision such as the coaching supervision client's well-being and development of the coaching supervision client using the stance outlined above. Other common topics mentioned above are explored in more detail in Chapter 14.

DOI: 10.4324/9781003390527-6

A Solution Focused Supervision Stance

Pragmatism and Curiosity

The SF approach is pragmatic in that it is goal oriented and practical, as it directs the focus towards generating possibilities in the direction of desired change versus interacting with the problem and focusing extensively on the origins and events leading to the problem. Solution Focus employs practical and concrete pathways to facilitate the desired outcome and helps supervision clients see tangible steps they can take to improve or manage the situation. While acknowledging and respecting the problem and the supervision client's point of view, we invite them to consider another perspective with evocative questions and a "tap on the shoulder" (Berg & de Shazer, 1994).

> Yes, I hear what a challenge this situation is for you. I'm curious. Suppose, it was one of those days where you had all the clarity and confidence you needed to handle this situation, what would you be doing, feeling and thinking, instead?

> Given what you know now, how would you manage that differently?

Interactional View

The origin of the SF approach is based on the interactional view that patterns are developed and change is experienced between people versus a belief that patterns and problematic issues reside within the individual. It is from this perspective that we invite the supervision client to view the situation. In the case supervision example provided below, the supervision client expresses concern that she is somehow inadequate or not knowledgeable about a certain topic. The supervisor explores the nature of the interaction between the supervision client and her client, as a means of processing the concerns and shifting the narrative away from a perceived deficit to a wider view of the interaction between the supervision client and their client, which facilitated a different perception. If problems occur interactionally, then solutions and improvements can occur interactionally. Instead of focusing on linear cause-and-effect in relationships, the interactional view considers circular causality. Solution Focus explores how patterns of interaction that are desired occur and highlights behaviours and interactions within a system are mutually influencing and reinforcing (Watzlawick et al., 1967). These shifting points of view can facilitate self-efficacy away from feeling stuck and powerless. We often view desired change as one that begins with the other person changing first or removing obstacles in the way of what is wanted. The interactional view suggests that change can be initiated by viewing a situation differently, approaching it differently or doing something differently, which in turns creates a different interactional pattern.

Progress (Not Explanation) Orientation

Instead of generating possible causes of and explanations for a difficulty or challenge, SF conversations generate possibilities towards the desired state and orient the supervision client towards the future focused solution narrative versus the problematic past narrative. This creates an alternate pathway to viewing the situation, and generates movement and progression, versus feeling stuck or hindered. The progress is anchored on the contractual agreement for supervision and what the supervision client wants from the session. Therefore, progress and movement occur as the focus is on making small steps in the desired direction.

Viewing Clients as Resourceful and Whole (Resource – Not Deficit Orientation)

One of the most important aspects of an SF supervisor is the general tenor and stance. The overall attitude is positive, respectful and hopeful (Dolan, 2024). The stance of the supervisor is based on key assumptions about the supervision client as having existing competencies, capabilities, resources, both internal and external, that can be utilised. In viewing the client through this lens, we are resource activators, which are important catalysts for change. When supervision clients are able to view themselves as capable and having self-efficacy, they become more motivated and hopeful in the change management process.

Respect (for Supervision Client and Their Client)

At the heart of SF thinking is the profound respect for the client, in honouring their way of thinking, their words, their views, their longings and best hopes. De Shazer had the ability to "simultaneously demonstrate respect and invite hope while using language carefully and intentionally" (de Shazer et al., 2021, p. 24). Our choice of words, text and desired direction embodies a desire to maintain the integrity of the supervision client's narrative, as "faithfully and respectfully as possible" (de Shazer et al., 2021, p. 24). The degree to which we attend to these details and honour the supervision client's perspective requires "attention, absorption, and disciplined focus" (de Shazer et al., 2021, p. 24). Not only does the SF supervisor assume the best about their supervision clients, they intentionally refrain from interpretations and explanations. Additionally, the SF supervisor seeks detailed descriptions from the supervision client about their ideas, ways of working, and how they managed. This heightens the sense of self-efficacy and sense of competence in their knowledge or intuition in solving their own dilemmas. It values and respects the supervision client as being resourceful and capable, in their past, their present and future.

One key factor in case supervision is to always talk about the client of your supervision client as if they were also in the room. This is important for several reasons:

- Maintaining respect for the client throughout the session
- Serving as a reminder to consider the client's perspective, beliefs, feelings and experiences to enhance the quality of support

- Encouraging reflective practice to process interactions, interventions or approaches that impact the client
- Promoting a sense of accountability in terms of their ethical and professional conduct
- Facilitating constructive feedback and guidance in relation to the supervision client-client relationship
- Maintaining confidentiality and respect of the client and what is/is not shared in supervision

Parallel Learning

Parallel learning is a process whereby the supervision client learns concurrently from sharing their experience as it relates to their client's situation, through shared experiences, observations and interactions. The supervisor can facilitate parallel learning by inviting the supervision client to reflect on the situation they have brought to supervision and explore what they have observed and learned from any similarities in what their client has brought to their coaching session. For instance, a supervision client expresses frustration and insecurities about how to deal with a client who is asking for advice, knowing that giving advice is not considered part of coaching, yet feels the pressure to deliver what their client is seeking. The supervision client then asks their supervisor what they should do, in essence asking for advice. The supervisor can explore this dilemma with the supervision client, by using the parallel learning process, and explore this several ways. The supervisor can explore what the supervision client has learned about themselves and about the situation and these reflections can also relate to the relationship the supervision client has with their client. Often what emerges is that the supervision client has gained some confidence in how they might deal with this situation and in turn has activated their own resources, and transfers this awareness to their own coaching situation.

Using Recordings in Case Supervision

Coaches who train with the International Coaching Federation will be used to recording their sessions and taking these to a mentor coach as part of their journey to becoming accredited or renewing their accreditation. The definition of mentor coaching is:

> Mentor Coaching for an ICF credential consists of coaching and feedback in a collaborative, appreciative and dialogued process based on an observed or recorded coaching session to increase the coach's capability in coaching, in alignment with the ICF Core Competencies
> (International Coach Federation, n.d.a)

Chapter 10 explores in detail what mentor coaching is, with an annotated transcript to show how the process works.

Table 6.1 Differences between ICF Mentor Coaching and Case Supervision With a Recording

ICF Mentor Coaching	Case Supervision with a Recording
Main goal: passing ICF performance evaluation or fulfilling renewal requirements	Main goal: personal and professional development of the coach, support and upholding ethical standards
Focus on concrete feedback related to minimum standard requirements of ICF	Focus on the expressed learning goals of the supervision client
Focus on doing coaching the ICF way	Focus on the "being" of the coach
Byproduct: personal development of the coach	Byproduct: growth in European Mentoring and Coaching Council (EMCC) standards/competency indicators and ICF competencies

Recordings of coaching sessions can also be brought to supervision although the focus is different. In case supervision the supervisor would invite the supervision client to state what learning they want to get from the recording, i.e. the focus is on the supervision client's professional goals rather than evaluation of whether they meet ICF core competencies. The supervisor would start by asking what went well in the session (getting specific details), and what the supervision client has already learnt about what they would do differently with the benefit of hindsight. They would then ask if it would be useful to offer their own reflections in relation to the learning goal of the supervisee. This is done using the SF stance outlined above of being curious, respectful and focusing on strengths. Ideas may also be offered in relation to what the supervision client could improve on, but handed back to the supervision client about what they want to do with the ideas offered. In some cases, it might be necessary for the supervisor to offer direct feedback for example the supervision client moving beyond the coaching role to a more consulting role without explicitly stating the reasons for this or partnering with their client, or when an ethical issue occurs but has not already been picked up by the supervision client.

See Table 6.1 for a summary of the differences between ICF mentor coaching and case supervision with a recording.

Example of Case Supervision With an Annotated Transcript

Below is an annotated transcript of a SF case supervision session illustrating the tenets described above.

Solution Focused supervision always starts with setting the agenda and asking what the coach's best hopes from the supervision are. While the coach immediately mentions a case to discuss, the supervisor notices the coach is ill, and links this to previous supervision sessions where the supervision client was exhausted. While the agenda normally comes primarily from the supervision client, the supervisor needs to be mindful of balancing the different functions of supervision (outlined in chapter 2, see pp. 7–27) and their role in checking in on the supervision client's wellbeing when this seems warranted. Here the supervisor first uses coping questions to identify strengths and resources and then partners with the coach to see if wellbeing would be a useful item to add to the agenda and explore more before coming back to the case.

Coaching supervision client:	I've got a case to discuss today but I'm ill, so apologies if I need to mute and cough.
Coaching supervisor:	You were saying before Christmas, you were super busy and exhausted. I was wondering, how have you been?
Coaching supervision client:	We moved house, which was stressful, but went really well. I had a week off, and that was lovely. Then I got back to work and got ill. I haven't slept for two weeks and am really exhausted. My client work is okay, but I'm forgetting things. A couple of big work deadlines are pending which are really stressful. And a close friend died before Christmas completely unexpectedly. He had a heart attack while driving. So it's been a bit of a roller coaster.
Coaching supervisor:	How are you coping?
Coaching supervision client:	The bereavement really knocked me for six because I've known him since I was a baby. So just going with it, allowing myself to cry. I talked to my manager and requested no new referrals until the new year and no bereavement work at the moment.
	I've managed to stop more things coming in. It's been really nice to get back to work and see my coaching clients. Because I've got so many things in my head, when I'm with clients, I can totally focus and be present. So it's actually weirdly relaxing to work and that's helping me cope.
Coaching supervisor:	What do you want from the supervision? Is there a need to attend to how you are and how you could strengthen yourself?
Coaching supervision client:	It might be helpful because I can't keep going like this; I am really tired. I have these two massive deadlines at the end of the month. So maybe how do I just get through the next couple of

	weeks because I don't want to slide down and not manage my commitments.
Coaching supervisor:	So how do you hang on and still keep your commitments?
Coaching supervision client:	Yes. I need to look after myself over the next couple of weeks.

Below is an example of a question where the supervision client is seen as resourceful and whole, it is assumed they already know about how to look after themselves and are invited to share to elicit existing strengths and resources before exploring what else might be needed.

Coaching supervisor:	What do you know about yourself and how you carefully look after yourself when it works?
Coaching supervision client:	Normally I exercise and I can't do that because I'm just coughing all the time. But I'm still eating well. I'm still trying to sleep. Actually the one thing that is really helpful is mindfulness. Every morning I wake up do a ten-minute breathing meditation or a body scan before I get the kids up, because normally my day would be about others. So I've turned the day around and I'm starting with me. I feel a bit more relaxed again, just going back to my routine. I'm very organised and efficient, I've got to do lists, I've got reminders in my phone. I'm prioritising what needs to be done today, what can wait, and not beating myself up. I can't function at my usual level, so I just do what I can.
Coaching supervisor:	You said, not beating yourself up. Is there a way of stating what you're doing instead of beating yourself up, that might be helpful to explore?
Coaching supervision client:	It's just being kind and talking to myself and saying it's okay. Like today I came home and felt physically drained. I had about ten things I could have done and I just went to lie down. So it's having breaks, but telling myself, this is okay. If you push yourself, it's going to be worse later. So stop now and then see how you feel. And trust I do always get things done.

As in coaching, supervision is always about partnering between the supervisor and supervision client. The supervisor partners here to check whether this is enough exploration or the supervision client wants to explore more.

Coaching supervisor:	Do you want to explore more around this or are you good with these kinds of explorations?
Coaching supervision client:	What if it doesn't work? What do I do if I notice it going down before I get to my deadlines?

The supervisor offers an alternative to the miracle question here, exploring the preferred future in terms of how the supervision client would notice themselves responding when they are their best self.

Coaching supervisor:	And how would you then like to respond if you are your best self, your kindest self?
Coaching supervision client:	I think asking for help earlier. I'm not always good at asking for help. Sometimes I just get cranky first and I could have just asked earlier. So noticing when I get irritable. Then reach out and say I need a break or I need help.
Coaching supervisor:	So noticing, asking for help. And the difference that's going to make?
Coaching supervision client:	If I get really irritable, either my husband or my kids will get irritable. And it just starts a really unhelpful spiral for all of us. If I could do my part to keep the house calm, it helps all of us and helps me.
Coaching supervisor:	Anything else on that that topic?
Coaching supervision client:	No that's good. Thank you.
Coaching supervisor:	As we were talking in the preparation, you said you'd had a case that you wanted to discuss?
Coaching supervision client:	So I've got this CEO that I've been seeing because I'm starting executive coaching, and I've seen him once. His HR recommended it. He had a 360 and got some feedback that he wasn't very happy with. He started work at this company before the pandemic so it's been a really difficult time. And he's actually done very well and grown the company. And now he's coming up for air and thinking, what do I do? There's just so many different parts of the case, and I can't see the woods for the trees and I don't really know what to do.

Any discussion about a case, always starts with the supervisor asking what the supervision client is looking for from the outcome of the discussion. As in all SF conversations, the coach's words and metaphors are used in the questions.

Coaching supervisor:	And if you did see the woods for the trees what would you be seeing?

Coaching supervision client:	Well, I think I'd have a much better understanding. We had a chemistry call, then we had one session and a lot of it was the getting to know you part. He talked about all this feedback and I suddenly realised I've been coaching for years, but am new to executive coaching, I don't know anything about these tools that he was talking about. And I didn't want to look stupid and go I don't know what this "red, green, blue, yellow" thing is. I've not heard of that. So I didn't understand that. I want to understand him and what's going on for him. But I also want to understand what's going on for me, because I was feeling very anxious about our second session. Then he cancelled because he got stuck on a business trip. I just felt huge relief which is not normally how I feel. I normally really look forward to seeing my coachees. So I just want to make sense of what's happening, what's about me, what's about him so that I can deal with the bit about me so I can be there for him and connect with him.

As outlined in chapter 3 (see pp. 27–42), SF supervision values pluralism and responsiveness to the particularities of context rather than applying generalities such as diagnosis. Here it would be easy to try and explore "what is really going on for the client" or indeed "what is really going on for the supervision client" in order to find the real problem and therefore correct solution. Instead the supervisor invites the coach to describe what their preferred outcome is in this situation.

Coaching supervisor:	And the not anxious part would be the looking forward to that. That's what you described as being the normal you?
Coaching supervision client:	Yeah so looking forward to it. But it's also being present, not getting distracted by feeling out of my depth, because this has taken me right back to when I started being a coach and going, what on earth am I doing? He's very intelligent, very articulate, wants to focus on results, wants things to happen quickly. I'm feeling intimidated by him. I want to find the empathy for him and be present. So I'm not distracted by all my stuff.

However as the coach goes back to mentioning "their stuff", the supervisor is respectful of this and partners with them to see how much this needs exploring, while explicitly linking that the exploration would be in service of moving forwards towards the preferred future, rather than in understanding for its own sake.

Coaching supervisor:	To what extent do we have to look at your stuff in order to do that?
Coaching supervision client:	I've done so much work on myself over the years and got over this" I'm not good enough" This has taken me straight back into it. So it might be helpful to think, how do I get out of it more quickly? Because I'm not in the same place as I was years ago, so I'm hoping this is just a temporary blip. He's a CEO, he's really important. And what do I know? I would like to get out of that.

The supervisor explores the supervision client's description of "imposter syndrome" as a theme in her life and how she interacts with this narrative. What emerges are alternative dialogues that the supervision client describes as alternative views and perspectives about her, rather than a reality of who she really is.

Coaching supervisor:	Do you have a name for the "that"? That you want to get out of?
Coaching supervision client:	I think that the traditional name is imposter syndrome. I'm a good coach, but I'm not an executive coach. I don't know about all of these assessment measures. I don't know some of the language he's using. So who am I to show up in this space? So yes that's what I would call it.
Coaching supervisor:	And what kind of relationship would you like with the imposter syndrome, in the best case?

The supervisor invites the client to "externalise" the problem. This is a move from narrative practice which allows a separation from "the person" from "the problem". When the client can see the problem as "out there" rather than as a part of themselves, they can usually find more ways of responding.

Coaching supervision client:	I'd like to just go. "Oh, here we go again. You're over this". Kind of have a bit of humour. Just go: "Okay. Thanks for reminding me to keep on my toes, but just go away". I can acknowledge it because there are some useful things that I want to learn about. I don't need to be bothered by it. But I really was in that session.

Coaching supervisor:	Go away, go away. And do you have an idea what the imposter syndrome might reply? If that's a useful game?
Coaching supervision client:	I want to keep the useful bit of it, you know, I don't know about these assessments. So that's why I would really like some information and advice from you, because I know you've done executive coaching. So that's another thing I'd like out of the conversation. But I don't know whether it would say, "but I'm just trying to remind you to do this" in a nice way or whether it would actually be, "but you really don't know what you're doing".
Coaching supervisor:	So when you're in it, it feels like it's real. What does the imposter syndrome see you think, feel or do that weakens its influence?
Coaching supervision client:	Well, the fact I'm bringing this up to supervision, the fact that I've spotted it earlier. That I can actually sit here and laugh about it; I can relate to it differently than I used to years ago. I'm just thinking back to how much progress that shows that I've made. I can actually say I am really good at what I do, I'm good at coaching and at being with people. I don't think he would have noticed that I didn't know any of this stuff. So how I showed up in the session was quite good and I asked lots of really nice SF questions. So all that's different.
Coaching supervisor:	And that difference is something that helps the imposter syndrome to say, okay. Bye bye.
Coaching supervision client:	Yes and I think I need to get some of the information and I need to have a plan – what is it I actually need to learn more about? Then I would be clearer and getting back on track quicker.
Coaching supervisor:	So it sounds like you're using the "be on your toes" good advice and just say that sounds factual to me. Is that a word you might use?
Coaching supervision client:	Yes I can challenge it factually. In the session, it did feel a bit like anxiety. But afterwards I was like. No. Here we go again. I can see it; which is better.

The supervisor asks for permission to share and then offers some ideas, but without attachment. The coach is left to decide what if anything is helpful to them. Edwards and Chen (1999) suggest that supervision clients' innate tendency to make their own progress is more likely to come to the fore when supervisors hold their own thinking lightly. This also fits with ICF core competency 7.11: Shares observations, insights and feelings, without attachment, that have the potential to create new learning for the client

(International Coach Federation, n.d.b)

Coaching supervisor:	Would it help if I shared a personal experience around issues like that?
Coaching supervision client:	Super helpful.
Coaching supervisor:	And you take what's useful and the rest just throw away. When I started as an executive coach I felt very similarly that I needed to know all these tools and these assessments. Then I started realising these are ever changing hypes and fads and it's like Insights one day and DISC the next day. There is no way you can possibly know all the assessments. Because different companies will do different assessments. I learned to not expect myself to know everything. Just know one. And then if somebody says well but we're working with a "blah blah blah". And then I say, is it something like the "bloop bloop bloop"? And they say, yeah, it's like that. So okay, can you give me some information? So I'm prepared to go back to HR and ask them to tell me. Because I think there is no way you can know or even need to know all of them. But I don't know What's your response? And please edit and reject.
Coaching supervision client:	That's really helpful thanks. I guess what I do need to know is even if I don't know the tool, what do I then do with it? He talked about having had this feedback which he agreed with. But with the tool, he was, I think, a "green" and "blue". He felt very boxed in by it and wanted to be more yellow, wanted to be more creative anyway. But then he was like "this is how I am". He was seeing this as a factual definition of himself. He could say, well, I can see this bit that I agree with, but I want to be over here and it's telling me I can't. So I wasn't really sure how to then follow it up.

It would be tempting for the supervisor to offer a solution about what the supervision client could have done. Instead the supervision client is asked for their perspective. As Pichot and Dolan state: 'The role of the solution focused supervisor is to pull the wisdom from the therapists rather than tell them what to do.'

(2003, p. 173)

Coaching supervisor:	What do you think about these kind of boxes?
Coaching supervision client:	I think that if somebody finds them useful, great. And if they don't, great. I've personally found some of them helpful but I take it with a pinch of salt by going what's useful from it? And so I'm very open to coachees – either way it doesn't matter. But he wasn't really open. I had asked him what if anything, was useful. And I said to him, we don't fit into nice boxes. It's more like it's a framework that helps some people. And if you find it helpful, great. But if you don't, we can throw it out the window. And I suppose the bit I found really difficult was he didn't like it, but he didn't want to throw it out the window either. And so we got a bit stuck.

When discussing any client in supervision, it is important to explore what progress or the preferred future would look like. As mentioned in chapter 3 (see pp. 27–42) this preferred future centres on the interaction between the supervision client and their client. This is different from many other models that may look to explore what was happening for the client here.

Coaching supervisor:	What's the outcome that you would like for him and for you in the coaching relationship?
Coaching supervision client:	Well, I want him to figure out what it is he wants from the coaching. I guess we started on that because it was the first session. He had some clear ideas.

Then we got bogged down by the tools. It's just helping him get the clarity on where he wants to go. I feel like if my imposter syndrome is not bothering me, I can be more present and be more open. I had so much going on in my head in the session. I'm used to coachees being stuck for all sorts of reasons, and I'm okay with that normally. I just want to feel that there's movement, that he's satisfied and that I'm showing up and being present in that process.

Coaching supervisor:	So if you're showing up and you're present and he says, well, but you know what I am blue and green so that means I can't be yellow, which I think that's where

the stuckness was, how would you respond to invite unstuckness?

Here the supervision client is invited to move from the more general preferred future to describe in more detail what they would be doing when they are showing up and present, even though the client is still stuck. The more detail they are able to describe, the greater the likely scale and momentum of change

(Iveson et al., 2012)

Coaching supervision client: I'd ask him whether it's helpful to keep talking about this tool.

Or do we set it aside and have a conversation as we were at the start of the session? I suppose it's inviting him to put it down. If he doesn't, saying what I'm hearing is that these are the bits you agree with and these are your strengths and this is what you want more of. Is that right?

Is that something you want to explore more in the session? Do you want more of this creativity? Not rushing. I think I was rushing thinking "I don't know this. I should know the answers". Let's just stay with this. Let's ask some questions. Some of them will land well, some won't. That's okay. Partnering "would you be open to me just asking some questions and see which one lands?" I don't think I did much of that in the session and actually, that's a sign of strength as a coach, not a weakness that I don't know what I'm doing.

As described in chapter 3 (see pp. 27–42), Thomas (2011) outlines three communication styles of the supervisor moving from more indirect to more direct communication: metaphor, semaphore and two by four. Here the supervisor offers a direct idea– that perhaps the supervision client can help the coachee question some of their beliefs about themselves or the tool – but again through tone of voice and use of the word maybe, this is not something the coach is being told to do but offered as a possible option.

Coaching supervisor: What springs up for me is there's stuckness that's kind of self-made.

And then there is stuckness that's a result of the tool being used in a not so helpful way, which is saying "if you are not yellow, you cannot ....." I mean, that's just a very limiting sentence.

Maybe that's also something to question in a coaching session: I don't believe that tool really means that. So maybe looking into the tool and saying, if you're not yellow now, it doesn't mean you can't ever be yellow.

Coaching supervision client: What sparked off when you were just saying that was I don't know where that idea came from, whether that was how it was presented. The whole company did it. And I don't know whether this was his idea or what HR was saying. That might be an interesting exploration of where did that idea come from and how useful is it?

Coaching supervisor: I mean, there's one way of looking at it and there's another way of looking at it. He's free with your invitation to interpret it any way he wants. Would you like to spend some more time on the coaching relationship with the executive, or should we also move into how can you find out the things that you want to find out, to feel that you've done your due diligence?

Here the supervisor partners with the supervision client to reflect on the supervision agreement and where they want to go next.

Coaching supervision client: Well, I've got a clearer idea. So I'm really liking that conversation about imposter syndrome. And that's enough to get me back on track. If I figure out what I need to learn, that will free me up to be with him, be flexible and come up with questions. So what do I need to go and learn about to feel more skilled because I do think there are things that I don't know that would be useful to read up about?

Coaching supervisor: I'm wondering, do you think you need to learn this, right now, or is there also an opportunity to just go with the flow and see? The way I went about it is basically just asking the HR department of that company, saying, I'm seeing you're using this tool. I'm generally familiar with personality assessments, and I just want to make sure that I understand it the way that you guys are using it. There is no way you can you know, it doesn't detract from your competence if you ask them. And then kind of build up your repertoire as you go along.

Coaching supervision client: I hadn't even thought of going to ask HR about it. I thought, I need to go and do some reading. So maybe it's not like I need to go and find out lots of factual information. Maybe it's more about the process of what do I need to take into account. But if there's anything that you've heard that you think you're not doing or you could do that would be helpful.

The coach is asking for direct feedback and the supervisor is happy to share. There is a myth that solution focused supervisors do not give direction but as Pichot and Dolan (2003, p. 171) clarify: "Effective supervisors must acquire the ability to determine when they need to provide information".

Coaching supervisor: I guess my strategy has always been to say, there are so many of these things around. And yes, I know quite a lot of them, but I've never had a negative experience of someone saying, but you should know this. They were always very happy to say, okay, you're interested in how we're doing things here and you're interested in our specifics. And the specifics are always more useful to me because that's what I really want to know. I want to know how are they using it, and what for what purpose, and what is the benefit that they're hoping to get? So I don't know if that might be a strategy for you.

Coaching supervision client: I suppose it's going back to that, not letting the imposter syndrome stop me asking questions because I don't want to look stupid, but actually that's a really nice way of doing it. I'm familiar with how these work, but how have you used it? How have you shared it? How have you done the feedback? Because obviously I'm sure lots of companies it's going to be different. Maybe what I need to do is just be open to what questions pop up and write them down and then so what do I need to do to tackle this question? I remember this being a psychologist, there's only so much that you could read about, and it's a pointless waste of time reading everything until you actually have a coachee where it's relevant and meaningful and the information makes sense. So that's probably a better strategy, have

	a journal somewhere of what questions pop into my head after a session, what do I then follow up. And I can also bring them here. That feels a good place to leave it. Thank you.
Coaching supervisor:	Would you like to summarise, or is there any other way you would like to close our session?
Coaching supervision client:	I think that's good. So coming up with questions, and then the being mindful of asking for help, that's my two big takeaways from today. So that's yeah really helpful. I'm fine to leave that there.
Coaching supervisor:	You know what? The ripples that has what resonates with me is this. Noticing when I'm not in a good spot and can be kind to myself. That's something that I think is very good for me to remember as well. So thank you for that session.

Conclusions

The SF stance in supervision reminds us that we do not need to be the subject matter expert on the topics or content our supervision clients bring to supervision. The "not-knowing" stance reminds us that this position allows us to remain curious about what the supervision client is seeking, as a result of their question or topic raised. There is a longing or desire behind the problem that they bring. As an SF supervisor, we bring our curiosity, respect and belief that our supervision client is resourceful and can find their way. The example provided in this chapter offers a parallel learning experience. Just like the coaching client wanted answers related to the assessment, the supervision client also wanted answers about what they did not know. In both scenarios, asking questions that evoke what is wanted beyond that leads to insight, creative ways to move beyond a sense of stuckness and also, the tolerance or comfort for living with ambiguity and acceptance of that.

Reflective Exercise

We invite the reader to reflect upon your role as a coaching supervisor and how you would facilitate learning with your coaching supervision client when they bring a coaching client case for review.

New areas for growth

- How would you frame the process in the service of the coaching supervision client's learning?
- What common topics do you encounter when supervising case discussions?

- How might you use some of the ideas offered in this chapter on the SF stance to facilitate learning and growth for your coaching supervision client?

Reflect on previous supervision sessions that went really well

- What questions did you ask to enhance their insights, reflections and development?
- How did you embody the SF stance?

References

Berg, I.K. & de Shazer, S. (1994). *A Tap on the shoulder: Six useful questions in building solutions*. Brief Family Therapy Center.

de Shazer, S., Dolan, Y., Korman, H., Trepper, T., McCollum, E., & Berg, I. K. (2021). *More than miracles: The state of the art of solution-focused brief therapy*. Routledge.

Dolan, Y. (2024). *Solution-focused therapy: The basics*. Routledge.

Edwards, J., K. & Chen, M. (1999) Strength-based supervision: frameworks, current practice and future directions. *The Family Journal: Counselling & Therapy for Couples & Families*. *17*: 349–357.

International Coach Federation. (n.d.a). Mentor Coaching. International Coach Federation. https://coachingfederation.org/credentials-and-standards/mentor-coaching

International Coaching Federation (n.d.b). *ICF Core Competencies*. https://coachingfederation.org/credentials-and-standards/core-competencies

Iveson, C., George, E., & Ratner, H. (2012). *Brief coaching, a solution focused approach*. Routledge.

Pichot, T., & Dolan, Y. M. (2003). *Solution-focused brief therapy: Its effective use in agency settings* (pp. 159–179). The Haworth Press Inc.

Thomas, F. N. (2011). Semaphore, metaphor, ... two-by-four. In T.S. Nelson (Ed). *Doing something different. Solution-focused brief therapy practices* (pp. 243–248). Routledge.

Watzlawick, P., Beavin, J. H., & Jackson, D. D. (1967). *Pragmatics of human communication: A study of interactional patterns, pathologies, and paradoxes*. W. W. Norton & Company.

7 Coaching Supervision With Clients Using Different Coaching Models/Approaches

Svea van der Hoorn and Kirsten Dierolf

Introduction

This chapter dives into how to respond as a coaching supervisor when invited to supervise a coaching supervision client who draws on a different coaching model/approach from those the coaching supervisor is familiar with and/or has expertise in. Solution Focused supervision with its emphasis on client goals and strengths and restraint when it comes to interpretations and advice is especially suited to collaborating with coaching supervision clients drawing from different models/approaches. This chapter offers some practical tips as well as a transcript of a session between a Solution Focused coaching supervisor and a coaching supervision client using transactional analysis.

The world of coaching is largely unregulated. There is a wide variety of approaches and models that coaches draw on in their work, which may then become part of what coaching supervisors find themselves engaging with during coaching supervision. Examples of models/approaches we have encountered include but are not limited to – GROW, systemic, transactional analysis, gestalt, family constellations, neuro-linguistic programming (NLP), ontological, integral, brain-based, neuroscience, trauma-informed, somatic, results, narrative, response-based and more.

Some coaching supervisors will make it explicit that they offer coaching supervision only to coaching supervision clients who draw on the same coaching models/approaches as those the coaching supervisor themselves has familiarity with. Some even specify that they will offer coaching supervision only on coaching models/approaches they have training in. This is not the stance of Solution Focused coaching supervision, although some Solution Focused coaching supervisors may prefer to offer coaching supervision to only those who coach from a Solution Focused approach.

How Are Coaching Models/Approaches Relevant in Coaching Supervision?

The European Mentoring and Coaching Council's (EMCC Global, 2019) coaching supervision competences refer to supporting the coaching supervision client to uphold professional standards. The following EMCC supervision

DOI: 10.4324/9781003390527-7

competences are seen as inviting coaching supervisors to draw on models and approaches:

EMCC Coaching Supervision Competence 2: Facilitates Development.
Enables the supervisee to improve the standard of their practice through a process of facilitated reflection.
EMCC Coaching Supervision Competence 3 Provides Support.
Provides a supportive space for the supervisee to process the experiences they have with clients and to prioritise their well-being as a coach or mentor.
EMCC Coaching Supervision Competence 5 Self-Awareness.
Consciously uses and develops the "self" in service of the supervision relationship and process.
EMCC Coaching Supervision Competence 6 Relationship Awareness.
Understands and works with the layers of relationship that exist in the supervision process.
EMCC Coaching Supervision Competence 7 Systemic Awareness.
Is able to recognise and work with the dynamics of human systems.

Whereas it might seem logical for coaching supervisors to make use of the vast ocean of online knowledge resources available to equip themselves to at least be familiar with a variety of coaching models/approaches, a Solution Focused coaching supervisor will likely take a different approach. In keeping with the stance that people are resourceful and that it is wise to start with what is already known and working well, the Solution Focused coaching supervisor may well start with questions such as these:

- I noticed in your email signature that you indicate you work in an XYZ coaching model/approach. How are you hoping we will make use of this expertise/training you already have in the coaching supervision that we will be doing together?
- I am aware you have decided to contract for a Solution Focused coaching supervision package with me. You let me know you have limited knowledge of Solution Focus but are keen to reflect on your coaching both through the models/approaches you already know, and the Solution Focused approach. Is now a good moment for us to discuss how you would like us to make use of coaching models and approaches in our work together?

Once it is established how the coaching supervision client would like to include reflecting on models/approaches in their coaching supervision, a Solution Focused coaching supervisor is less likely to head to the internet to research the models/approaches they are unfamiliar with and more likely to continue the conversation with an invitation like:

- "What if any resources would you like us to both refer to when reflecting on the models/approaches that you draw on in your work?"

Agreement is then reached that the coaching supervision client will bring to sessions the content about the model/approach that they wish to draw on. The coaching supervisor may agree to watch video clips, peruse a website or read an article as preparation for a coaching supervision session when requested to do so by the coaching supervision client. The purpose is not to gain expertise, but rather that the coaching supervisor and the coaching supervision client can collaborate by drawing on shared information. Here are a few examples that we received from coaching supervision clients:

- *The Complete Handbook of Coaching*, 3rd Edition (Cox et al., 2014)
- *The Handbook of Knowledge-Based Coaching: From Theory to Practice*, 1st Edition (Wildflower & Brennan, 2011)
- *International Journal of Evidence Based Coaching and Mentoring*, 2023, Special Issue 17

Exploration of these chosen resources opened conversations around what appealed to the coaching supervision client about their chosen model/approach, what the roles and responsibilities of the coach and the coaching client are, what are considered to be the necessary mechanisms of change and signs of progress in the particular coaching approach and more. Topics collaboratively reflected upon for each model/approach selected by the coaching supervision client as relevant to the coaching supervision include:

- What is the theory of change?
- Where and when does change happen?
- Is change something that happens inside or outside the person? Is it interactional or intrapsychic?
- What are the search spaces that are privileged in the models?

Figure 7.1 is an illustration which guides Solution Focused coaching supervisors in conversations about the possible search spaces of different models/approaches.

Solution Focus differs from other approaches in that it looks at people in interaction rather than at inner mechanisms. You could say that we take the psycho out of psychology. As a social constructionist approach, Solution Focus is interested in the emergence of new identities rather than understanding (in our words "constructing") the old. This does not mean that Solution Focused coaching supervision is past allergic or avoidant. On the contrary, the past search space is routinely given time in coaching supervision as the space in which resourcefulness of the coaching supervision client is illuminated when asked for accounts of coping or success stories. Figure 7.2 shows how coaching supervisors can both respect wherever their coaching supervision client is at as they introduce what they are looking for from coaching supervision and also invite the conversation to move towards possibility talk and future growth.

	Search space for explanations	Search space for progress
Search space for resources	Positive Psychology	Solution Focused Questions
Search space for deficits	Psychoanalysis	Quality Management

Figure 7.1 Possible search spaces of different models/approaches
(Image by Kirsten Dierolf)

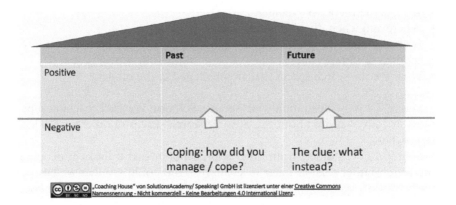

Figure 7.2 Coaching house: invite into the first floor
(Image by Kirsten Dierolf)

What Is Being Asked of the Coaching Supervisor?

Frank Thomas (2013) sheds light on what is being asked of the Solution Focused coaching supervisor when engaging with a coaching supervision client who describes their work and what they want from coaching supervision in what might be called "model/approach" talk. He points to the paradox and hence a tension to hold lightly, between adopting a not knowing, non-hierarchical stance, while simultaneously fulfilling the role of providing quality assurance guidance due to the coaching supervisor's greater expertise. The coaching supervisor is faced with moment-to-moment decisions about locating themselves in the role of gatekeeper, guide or guru (see Chapter 5, pp. 59–75 for more details).

Let's suppose a coaching supervision client brings as a topic "how do I work with the negative limiting beliefs of my coaching client? I don't think progress is possible until these have been dealt with".

Here is a short overview of how we notice other approaches conceptualising and dealing with "limiting beliefs", followed by a Solution Focused alternative. "Limiting beliefs" are mentioned in many psychotherapy models/approaches and also in the coaching methods that are based on them (Boden et al., 2012).

Cognitive behavioural therapy might treat "limiting beliefs" under the heading of a "cognitive distortion", a thought that someone holds which is not true. Cognitive distortions may be unconscious, not known to the client. The task of the therapist is to identify the distortion and make the client aware of it, so that the client can then change the belief or distortion that is the obstacle to becoming better. The position of the therapist here is one of an observer and maybe also of an analyser. When the therapist has identified a cognitive distortion which is unknown to the client and the client does not agree that it is a "distortion" but thinks that their belief is true, the client can become "resistant" in the eyes of the therapist. In Solution Focused coaching, we would not take the stance of an objective observer but rather do our best to collaborate with the client. We would think that if we think the client is "resistant", we are in the wrong and need to work on listening more closely.

Albert Ellis' Rational Emotive Behaviour Therapy (The Albert Ellis Institute, n.d.) also uses the concept of "limiting beliefs" and even has a nice mnemonic for it: ABC, an activating trigger (A) for the false belief (B) and the consequences (C) that flow from the false belief. Understanding the activating trigger and coming to a new belief is recommended as a course of action for the therapist. In Solution Focus, we would not go looking for "activating triggers". Rather than asking for the story of the trigger (which is usually linked to the problem description), we would invite the client to speak about their responses to the problem, instances in which they were able to act like they want to act and then explore and expand these.

NLP is based on the analysis of inner human structures as they present themselves in language. Dilts (1990) identifies five levels of inner organisation:

1 environment and external constraints,
2 behaviour,
3 mental maps and strategies defining capabilities,
4 capabilities organised by belief systems and
5 beliefs organised by identity.

An NLP practitioner can identify limiting beliefs by the language a client uses. For example, the client may be using presumptive language, language which "hides" a presupposition, e.g. "I don't have time to go to the gym" hides the presupposition that time is the limiting factor and not, for example, prioritisation. Challenging the presupposition might help the client see that they have more agency in the matter than they thought they had. Solution Focus would assume that the client has good reasons to think the way they think and rather than challenging the presupposition would invite the client to "suppose you had more time", for example. Also, the Solution Focused coaching supervisor would not look at the person as an individual in control of their inner workings but rather view coaching supervision clients as embedded in relationships which contribute to what they think about themselves.

Solution Focus does not believe in "limiting beliefs". A "belief" is an unjustified reification, something that is made into a thing by language, which is not a thing. A "belief" is something that is observed from the outside and shows in a person's action. For example, if you believe that there is some birthday cake left, you will go to where cake is usually kept, fully expecting to find it there. After all you put it there after your party yourself. What you did not know was that I had a late night snack attack and ate the leftover cake. That you had planned to offer it the next day to guests was unknown to me and not part of our communication. Concluding that I am a greedy, inconsiderate person who cannot be trusted would be a faulty belief. The alternative is to conclude that there has been a failure in our communication. Rather than go look "into" the human being, Solution Focused coaching supervisors would focus on the interactions and descriptions of preferred realities.

Some examples of situations in which other approaches would identify a "limiting belief":

- I don't deserve …
- I am not strong enough for …
- I am too old for …
- I will never be able to …

Ways of working with situations like this in a Solution Focused or social constructionist way would be:

Accepting That This Is What the Client Thinks Right Now

We would not argue with the person and rather respect their description. We then might explore what kind of relationship they would prefer with this statement. Do they want to explore what they would like to believe instead? Would they like to prove that statement wrong? Is it sometimes even a helpful statement that they may want to retain (or parts of which they want to retain)?

Exploring the Preferred Future

We might ask "Suppose you had the relationship with the statement that you prefer, what might that look like? What might you be noticing that is different?

About you? About your interactions with others? About the way they respond to you?" We would ask for a detailed description of who would notice what and what the interactions might look like.

Coaching supervision client:	I would like to feel I deserve more respect.
Coaching supervisor:	Suppose you felt you had that respect, what would be the first sign that would tell you?
Coaching supervision client:	When I speak at professional meetings, my colleagues would listen to my presentation of the case.
Coaching supervisor:	And what might become possible for you then?
Coaching supervision client:	I would be able to do justice to the way I coach and not get railroaded by their suggestions about working in a different model.
Coaching supervisor:	And what might your colleagues begin to notice about you when you are able to do justice to the way you coach?
Coaching supervision client:	They would see that I am serious about how I go about the coaching I do, and would ask me questions about my way of working instead of telling me how to coach the client in their model.
Coaching supervisor:	And how would you let them know that you prefer them to ask you questions about your model/approach?
Coaching supervision client:	Hmmm, I'd have to stop being so frustrated and let them know that while I value their contributions, the questions that invite me to get really clear on how to coach well in my model are the most useful.

Exploring Instances of the Preferred Future Already Happening

Talking with coaching supervision clients about instances in the past is focused on moments where they already experienced themselves thinking, feeling and acting in the ways they described as what they want instead. These instances may contain valuable hints with which to build improvements in their standard of practice. Exploring these instances in rich detail paints a different picture of who the coaching supervision client is and opens new ways of thinking about the coaching supervision client for both.

What many Solution Focused coaching supervisors say is that Solution Focus keeps them in the role of a partner of the client. They centre the coaching supervision client and collaborate with them. They are not analysing or thinking that they know something more about the coaching supervision client or about the coaching clients, than the coaching supervision client knows.

Solution Focused Coaching Supervision in Action with a Coaching Supervision Client Who Draws Explicitly on a Specific Model

In the following transcript of a coaching supervision session, we invite you to notice the following that are characteristic of Solution Focused coaching supervision. When and how does the coaching supervisor demonstrate:

- pragmatism and curiosity,
- interactional view,
- orientation towards progress rather than towards explanation and understanding,
- viewing clients as resourceful and whole by adopting a resource not deficit orientation and
- respect – for both the coaching supervision client and their coaching client as described in the coaching supervision conversation.

Coaching supervisor: [00:00:14:18] Thank you for coming in for coaching supervision. What are you bringing to our session today?

Coaching supervision client: [00:00:56:18] I'm glad to be here, and I've become aware that I'm getting in my own way with a client because of how I experience this client in our coaching sessions. At first, I was quite amused by myself and by what was happening. But I'm beginning to realise that it's now the second session where this has happened. And I thought, I need to bring this to supervision because I don't feel I'm doing a good enough job with the client.

Coaching supervisor: [00:01:33:25] Okay. And what kind of better job or different experience are you looking for?

Coaching supervision client: [00:01:40:07] Well, what I'm experiencing in myself is – I like to reflect using the Transactional Analysis model – I experience myself as wanting to go into my Free Child and sort of poke him in the ribs and not take him too seriously. And I already have an irreverent sense of humour, but he is very earnest about what he's talking about. In the way that he speaks, I experience him in his Parent ego state. He comes across as very in a way not judgemental, but quite sure that his way is the right way. There is only a mild amount of openness. And he's a leader of a team and that's what he wants to work towards. I

would like to do a better job at being his coach in my full awareness and not sliding around into other parts of my own ego states in relation to what I experience him as doing. So if I was his buddy I could joke with him. But as his coach, I don't think it's appropriate, even though it's very tempting.

Coaching supervisor: [00:02:56:27] I mean, as you aware, I'm a Solution Focused coaching supervisor and I'm not very well versed in Transactional Analysis. I hope that doesn't stop us from helping you make progress ... I'm wondering ... there's a difference between what you were just calling Free Child and Parent ego state and the interaction that makes possible and the coach and your full awareness, I think you termed it, and the interaction that being there makes possible. Would it be useful to talk a little bit about what the different interaction would be if you were more in your full awareness Coach Self?

Coaching supervision client: [00:03:43:18] Yes, because that's what I really desire. And, thank you for also saying that Transactional Analysis (TA) is unknown to you because then I'm aware and maybe you can just ask me if I use jargon words that are clear to me but don't mean anything to you?

Coaching supervisor: [00:04:00:00] Yes I will

Coaching supervision client: What you've already said is helpful because full awareness in TA terms would be being in my Adult ego state. And if I were in my Adult ego state, I would be aware of what I've just said to you, but I would be able to respond to the client with that full awareness, rather than being reactive, I suppose. Your question has helped me to figure out it's not that I want to put aside my awareness of what's going on and what's happening in the interaction space. It's that I'd like to be able to be more deliberate, maybe in choosing how I'm responding to him rather than having this feeling, I'm just going to blurt things out. So because I have this feeling, I'm going to blurt things out, I then notice that I'm becoming more and more quiet and he's just telling stories. I think because he thinks that he needs to describe it more to me. So if you

	talk about the interaction, I'm certainly aware of that. So thank you. My holding back because I don't quite know what else to do is inviting him to tell more and more stories, which just makes me more and more amused. So it's actually making it worse, my keeping quiet. But I'm not quite sure how I could respond differently.
Coaching supervisor:	[00:05:40:13] And is this what you're looking for in our session today ... finding ways of how you could respond differently that transcend the I'm calling it dynamic, but I don't know if there's a better word for it?
Coaching supervision client:	[00:05:55:21] Interaction is fine. Yeah. When I heard you say that word, it was really helpful because I thought that's it's the between us that I'm struggling with. I'm not really struggling with knowing what I'm experiencing and how that fits with my TA awareness, but I'm not translating that into something in my coaching conversation with him.
Coaching supervisor:	[00:06:16:19] Okay. So also there is an idea that your TA experience can really be helpful as at vantage point to look from (coaching supervision client nodded their head)? Okay. And by the end of our session, if you have some way of translating what you know into how you could respond differently, that would be useful?
Coaching supervision client:	[00:06:46:24] That would be excellent. Even if it's something that I am just going to experiment with. Because I'm very clear that anything would be better than me being quiet and him just telling more and more and more stories. And it does feel like a dereliction of duty. So while I'm saying this with a smile on my face, I do feel the responsibility as his coach to optimise my invitations to him, so that the work that we're doing together really takes him where he wants to go and not just that I sit there quietly being stuck.
Coaching supervisor:	[00:07:24:24] Yeah ... I must say, I'm very impressed with how aware you are of what you're experiencing and how aware you are of the different possibilities that exist. So I'm very happy to explore that with you. Do you have a preferred way of going about exploring this?

Coaching supervision client:	[00:07:50:07] That's a useful question. Let me think. I'm not I'm not a pros and cons person and I'm not an options person much. I think I'm quite an imagination person. And when I can see or imagine myself using myself more fully, that often helps me. So if you could help me somehow see myself being different with this man, that feels like a good way to go.
Coaching supervisor:	[00:08:27:05] So in Solution Focus, we have these future focused type of questions where I would ask you to imagine being in this state that you want to be as a fully aware coach, and then just exploring in your imagination what that would look like, what the interaction would look like and how your client would respond and how you would respond. Is that something I might invite you to try?
Coaching supervision client:	[00:08:53:29] That's so cool, because that's Free Child energy in TA terms. So that would allow me to use this energy I'm experiencing, but towards what I'm asking for. Yeah. So that's great. Thank you. That sounds good.
Coaching supervisor:	[00:09:16:09] Okay, so dear Free Child, can I invite you to play?
Coaching supervision client:	[00:09:24:12] I'm quite a serious Free Child, so I will keep my serious hat on as well.
Coaching supervisor:	[00:09:30:14] Yeah, okay. Suppose you are in your full awareness as a Parent ego state coach. And you are experiencing yourself as you want to be experiencing yourself in the coaching session. When would be the first moment in that coaching session that you'll notice that you're in this kind of different state?
Coaching supervision client:	[00:09:59:23] Ah … And by the way, that's called the Adult ego state.
Coaching supervisor:	[00:10:02:19] Adult ego state, okay.
Coaching supervision client:	[00:10:04:10] I don't want to get into my Parent with him.
Coaching supervisor:	[00:10:05:29] Okay. Sorry.
Coaching supervision client:	[00:10:07:07] No, that's fine. It's good for me to clarify that as well. Okay, so how would I be? The first moment? Hmm. Okay. I think the first moment is that I would notice it before we even begin our session.
Coaching supervisor:	[00:10:24:24] Mm hmm.

Coaching supervision client:	[00:10:26:07] Yes, I would. And that's something I'm not doing at the moment. So there we go. I would engage with myself about I know that I have this energy … and my question to myself would be how would I like to use this energy, but to use it in a full awareness way. And that might alert me that I need to listen to what he is truly wanting to see change and stop listening so much with amusement to the story that he tells. Ah. There we go. With my full awareness I would focus more on the man that he is, his vulnerabilities yes, and his desire to be doing a good job with his team. That would be my focus – who he wishes to be with them. Not who he is, which is what the story is that he's telling at the moment. Okay. So I would remember that my job is to invite him to talk about how he would like to become, and less talk about how he understands why he's being as he is at the moment.
Coaching supervisor:	[00:11:54:26] I have an observation. May I share?
Coaching supervision client:	[00:11:57:20] Sure.
Coaching supervisor:	[00:11:59:17] It sounds to me like what you're describing now is kind of also what's happening here with us.
Coaching supervision client:	[00:12:06:25] Oh, ok say more.
Coaching supervisor:	[00:12:09:11] You're saying you would like to help him to focus more on who he wants to become. And we are also talking about who you want to become in relationship to him. And it might be that that really shifts the interaction. I'm not sure if that speaks to you or not?
Coaching supervision client:	[00:12:33:26] That does. And what is coming into my mind is, I need to look at him more, to see him as the man that he is and stop just listening to the way that he uses language, which is quite pejorative. I'm suddenly beginning aware of what it is that is inviting me to miss seeing him in his fullness. He's got a way of taking you know, he says "the girls in my team" and I kind of go, Oh, that's an interesting word. And then I want to poke him and go, "Do you really call them girls to their faces?" Because that would be inappropriate in his workplace. I know that.

And he even knows that. But he just keeps doing it. OK So I think that's another thing I would need to be looking more at him and not listening to the commentary in my head, which is what's distracting me. And I can hear in my head things like "I wonder what they think when he says girls to them", because I know that this workplace doesn't support those kinds of ways of speaking. There's quite a culture of using language which is quite neutral in this workplace rather than pejorative. I'm distracted by that. So I'm thinking I would need to focus my full awareness on where he wants to go and not be so much listening to my immediate responses to where he is at the moment.

Coaching supervisor: [00:14:29:03] And how do you imagine he might respond to that?

Coaching supervision client: [00:14:32:22] Hmm. I think. Look, I can't know, obviously, but I think there's more chance that he would be able to explore with me to find his way of dealing with what for him is quite strange. He's been a leader for about ten, 15 years already. He came from an era where speaking in this way was completely fine. He sees himself as much more of a manager, not a leader. He is good at giving instructions and is well enough liked because he smiles a lot. So if I shifted in this way, I think that he might get an opportunity to explore territory which I had not realised is significant. He probably feels really vulnerable because I don't think that he has the lived experience of how to speak appropriately in this politically correct environment. It's not known to him.

Coaching supervisor: [00:15:39:27] Okay. Okay. And then this "not known" might lead to making fun?

Coaching supervision client: [00:15:50:00] Yeah. What I can see in my imagination is instead of it being me and him either bantering, we would suddenly be alongside. And he would be looking to where he wants to go with a sense of me being a supportive partner that has respect for the fact that it's a big challenge for him. And maybe at the moment he doesn't experience me as respecting the fact that it is a big challenge for him. I suddenly realise that from a TA point of view, it would be, he might be seeing me in a sort of Critical Parent positive way, which is, well: "she clearly knows how to do this. And I don't really want to reveal too much about that, I don't know how to do this". because the fact that I can joke about it makes me sound like I'm an expert at this.

Coaching supervisor: [00:16:48:27] And instead?

Coaching supervision client: [00:16:52:02] Well, instead, I would like him to experience that. I respect the fact that, the change in his team from being a team with men and women into for the first time ever, he is leading a fully female team with some very assertive women. Um. And that he's having to do business as usual with his team whilst actually trying to teach himself how to work with a group of people that he really doesn't have experience of how to manage and lead. I hadn't realised that until this conversation. Now that I'm putting bits together, from what he has said about the changes that have been happening in his organisation, I think I've been under-responsive to the context in which he finds himself. And thinking this is all his personal stuff.

Coaching supervisor: [00:17:54:17] Okay. And if you take the context perspective and take everything together, you in the Adult state, full awareness, aware of what's going on, plus aware of the context. What's emerging for you now about how you might respond next time you coach this person?

Coaching supervision client: [00:18:21:13] I'm smiling because the first thing that came to my mind as I heard you say that was "I owe him an apology". Yeah. And, you know, whether I decide to give him an apology literally in the coaching session or whether I just hold the apology, the apology energy in myself is fine. I can figure that out for myself. But. I think that my beginning would be more focused on where does he want to go? And maybe I might do something that I experienced you doing with me. Which is to offer him some observation about the challenge that he faces. I think what could be better than an apology is to give him a glimpse that I carry an awareness that this is challenging for him and to perhaps start my next session with: In the light of all of that, what is it that I've missed that he would like to add. So he can correct me. What are his thoughts about what we still need to add to our common understanding of where he wants to go. Because as soon as we do have a common understanding, from a TA point of view, we would be an Adult to Adult transaction. We would stop being in this wobbly kind of Parent-Child game. So I think that would be wise and would also fulfil my sense of it's my duty to open the space as the coach in a way that he can be functional and move towards his desired future. I haven't been doing that well enough. So I think that could be a significant improvement.

Coaching supervisor: [00:20:27:10] Mm hmm. Mm hmm. Do you want to go explore this a little more, or do you think we're almost complete with looking at this better future?

Coaching supervision client: [00:20:37:23] Yeah. Look, I think. I think we're almost complete and maybe even complete. So maybe let me just think to myself. Is there anything more? I have a different starting point. I have a place to step from into the session. And. I must just remember to do that. I can see us having a different conversation if I come into it in a different way. It's not guaranteed, I know that. But I think it's enough as an option. Yeah.

Coaching supervisor: [00:21:27:06] Would it be useful for us to spend a little bit of time around how you can pick yourself up if you're invited into this Parent-Child kind of game I think you called it in your TA model?

Coaching supervision client: [00:21:48:06] Yeah, well exactly. Ta has lots of nice words, "rackets and games" and things like that. But "games", yes. I'd like to just explore or figure out how can I remind myself of what I'm talking about here, because life gets busy. I'm also thinking about that when I'm due to see him next, it's towards the end of the day and I've got quite a lot on my plate in that day. So it's easy to just fall into the next session. And not take the value from this conversation.

Coaching supervisor: [00:22:38:20] Yeah. So how to remind yourself?

Coaching supervision client:	[00:22:41:10] Yeah. Yeah. And then maybe if I slide, how to remind myself.
Coaching supervisor:	[00:22:51:08] How do you generally remind yourself of things?
Coaching supervision client:	[00:22:55:14] Yeah. I'm thinking I need to put it in the appointment. I need to find myself like a code word or image and put that next to his name. And what comes to mind, it's something about smiling … yeah. There we go. Not smiling at him, but smiling with him. The more I think about this, the more I'm not smiling with him. So maybe smiling with him. I could just do two faces, but both with smiles on their faces instead of my face only, I don't know. Something like that. And the other thing is the word "vulnerability". I think I need to write that next to the appointment. Because I think I've been missing the fact of his sense of vulnerability. So I've been seeing him as if he's okay with all of this and he thinks they're not okay. But actually, I think this conversation has helped me to tune into the fact that he's probably on quite unsteady ground. Yeah. So I think that would be sufficient. I'll put two little smiling faces and the word "vulnerability". In fact I'm going to do that now. Just give me a minute (pauses while writing happens). Okay, that's good. That's good. And then you said if I slipped, if I found myself with all my good intentions evaporating?
Coaching supervisor:	[00:24:40:19] and only if that's likely to happen, I don't know.
Coaching supervision client:	[00:24:44:18] Look, I'm human. So of course it's likely to happen. I might have to use my apology idea. Direct communication is one of my skills. And, it's one of my strengths and capacities to say things to people and stay right on the contact boundary with them. And I think I might, if it were to start happening, it might be an opportunity to actually just say "what's happening in this moment". I haven't offered him that. And there's no good reason. I've got no evidence that he wouldn't appreciate that. I don't know why I haven't done that. But there we go. It doesn't really matter why. I think that's what, that's what I would like – to be bold,

because my way of being respectful to clients, in relation to their vulnerability is in fact to be bold and show my own vulnerability. Because I can see that it could add value to the situation. And then wait and see what he wants to do with it. Yeah. And then I can hear one of my trainers in my head going, "That's a closed question. Don't ask closed questions".

Coaching supervisor: [00:26:25:11] Oh, but it's a partnering question. Go ahead and tell them "shush".

Coaching supervision client: [00:26:27:29]. Yeah. Because I do think that respect is about the client choosing. But having the material to be able to make the choice otherwise, how can you? So that's also useful for me to be reminded that I mustn't pull back when I hear myself about to ask a closed question. I need to encourage myself to offer the closed question as a choice giver. And not listen to this voice, but to my own voice.

Coaching supervisor: [00:26:59:28] I'm super impressed how you're pulling in all of your awarenesses and knowledge to really help this client. And at the same time observing what's going, kind of being in the interaction in the most possible, possibly positive way. And at the same time, kind of looking at the interaction, to have an awareness about and a partnership around what would be the best form of interaction. So. Wow. Thank you. Anything else we need to do today?

Coaching supervision client: [00:27:39:06] No, I think that's. I think I can experience it in myself that I have more quietness. Before I was observing things and not being in it. And I feel that I found my location to be more in it with him and let my amusement about a topic which I think is very big for many people, is this political correctness in the workplace – how to get that right, But to let that sort of interest or amusement sit more quietly and rather bring more of myself back into the coaching, which is to be together with him, That's what I think had gone a bit wrong. I've become more of an observer in the session, rather than a full participant.

Coaching supervisor: [00:28:38:24] Wow, thank you for sharing this. I look forward to when we next meet.

Reflective Exercise

- Reflect on [00:08:27:05] to [00:10:24:24].

  What did you experience when the coaching supervision client corrected the coaching supervisor's accuracy of the model/approach terminology? How might you have responded?
- Reflect on [00:11:54:26] to [00:14:29:03]

  Notice how the coaching supervisor keeps the theme of imagining alive in the conversation. How might you have responded during this sequence?
- Reflect on [00:21:48:06] to [00:22:51:08]

  How might you have responded to this? What are your thoughts about using or not using concepts and language from a model/approach that you are not at home with?

References

Boden, M. T., John, O. P., Goldin, P. R., Werner, K., Heimberg, R. G., & Gross, J. J. (2012). The role of maladaptive beliefs in cognitive-behavioural therapy: Evidence from social anxiety disorder. *Behaviour Research and Therapy, 50*(5), 287–291.

Cox, E., Bachkirova, T. & Clutterbuck, D.A. (2014). *The complete handbook of coaching* (3rd Ed). SAGE.

Dilts, R. (1990). *Changing belief systems with NLP*. Meta Publications.

EMCC Global. (2019). *Supervision competence framework*. Retrieved from https://www.emccglobal.org/leadership-development/supervision/competences/

The Albert Ellis Institute. (n.d). *Rational emotive behaviour therapy*. The Albert Ellis Institute. Retrieved March 30, 2023, from http://albertellis.org/rebt-cbt-therapy/

Thomas, F. N. (2013). *Solution-focused supervision: A resource-oriented approach to developing clinical expertise*. Springer.

Wildflower, L., & Brennan, D. (Eds.). (2011). *The handbook of knowledge-based coaching: From theory to practice*. John Wiley & Sons.

8   Deliberate Practice

*Jane Tuomola, Kirsten Dierolf
and Svea van der Hoorn*

Introduction

Scott Miller, Mark Hubble and Daryl Chow (2020) have popularised Deliberate Practice as a way to improve therapeutic effectiveness. This chapter introduces ways in which coaching supervisors can support their coaching supervision clients to implement and use principles and practices from Deliberate Practice to improve their coaching capability. Coaching supervision clients start by collecting a baseline of feedback from their coaching clients in the form of an adapted session rating scale (SRS) (Miller et al., 2002) and an adapted outcome rating scale (ORS) (Miller & Duncan, 2000). The coaching supervisor then supports them to analyse the feedback and to plan improvement experiments and actions. The chapter first describes the theory of Deliberate Practice and then offers practical steps the coaching supervisor can take with their coaching supervision clients, as well as exploring how to improve their own effectiveness, both as a coach and as a coaching supervisor.

Recognising Good Coaching

Recognising that you are getting better at coaching can be difficult. You would need to define what good coaching is in general. As coaching is a very context dependent and complex activity, it is hard to discern whether you are a good coach or whether you are getting better at coaching in general. Somewhat more feasible is to discern improvement of your coaching in relation to a particular client in a particular context. It is also questionable whether a coaching supervisor can support coaches to develop "in general". Coaching supervision always needs to be attuned to the development goals of the specific coaching supervision client. Here are some of the criteria that may tell coaches that they are growing as a coach. You can see from the variety of these growth signals that it would be misguided to assume that a coaching supervisor could superimpose a coach-maturity linear trajectory, or typical stages of development mindset in relation to goodness of coaching (Hermel-Stanescu, 2015):

- Signs of a good coach include self-awareness
- Signs of a good coach include capacity to inspire others.

DOI: 10.4324/9781003390527-8

- Signs of a good coach include ability to build learning and growth facilitating relationships.
- A good coach displays flexibility, openness and a future orientation.
- A good coach is disciplined and respects work boundaries.

Allied fields such as psychotherapy and social work have been researching outcomes and effectiveness for many years, as well as looking into what supports practitioners in becoming more effective. Some relevant literature is shared below to offer insights into how coaches can improve their practice, and how coaching supervisors can support this process.

What We Can Learn From the Outcomes and Effectiveness Research in Allied Fields

Like coaching, counselling and psychotherapy are modalities characterised by conversation as the medium for creating change and improvement in client's lives. The field of psychotherapy has been researching outcomes for many years as well as what helps therapists become more effective. The overall effect size compared to untreated samples is about 0.8, meaning that the average psychologically distressed person who receives psychotherapy will be better off than 80% of those who do not make use of psychotherapy. However, psychotherapy as a field has not improved over time and these figures have stayed the same over many years (Rousmaniere et al., 2017).

What is interesting, and perhaps disconcerting, is that when asked individually by psychotherapy supervisors most therapists say they are improving over time. The data however does not support this. Goldberg and colleagues (2016) carried out the largest study to date on the impact of experience on treatment outcomes. They collected data from 175 therapists over 17 years and found not only did therapists not improve, but their average therapy results worsened over time. The research controlled for numerous factors including the severity of client problems, and how long clients stayed in therapy. One of the reasons given for these results is automaticity, that is, where what was initially done with a lot of mental energy is done with barely a thought. As beginner therapists gain experience, the process of therapy becomes more automatic and less deliberate. The downside of this is that once actions become more automatic it is harder to make specific intentional adjustments to them. Purposefully counteracting this automaticity is what lies at the heart of Deliberate Practice.

A research study was designed to explore the role of Deliberate Practice in the development of highly effective therapists, in particular, what these top performing therapists did outside the therapy room, i.e. before and after they saw clients (Chow et al., 2015). They found that highly effective therapists spent 2.5 times more time in Deliberate Practice before and after their sessions than average therapists. When they asked the therapists for a self-assessment of current effectiveness, the least performing therapists rated themselves at least as effective as the top performing therapists. What distinguished top performing therapists was what they were working on outside the therapy room. Three things were important: (1) ongoing measurement of one's results; (2) continuous identification of specific errors and targets for improvement; and (3) development, testing and successive refinement of new ways of working (Goldberg et al., 2016).

Research into the effectiveness of social work, another modality characterised by conversational practice, raises further questions about outcomes and effectiveness measurement. Cree et al. (2018) support the importance of monitoring outcomes and effectiveness for pragmatic and ethical reasons. "Evaluating effectiveness is of primary concern to social work practice; resources will always be limited, and those using services deserve the best". They go on to point to a paradox, namely, "evaluating effectiveness sits uncomfortably between new public management's (NPM's) imperative for measurement and efficiency within a market economy and agencies' own need to reflect on their practice and respond to the views of their service users. Such processes force agencies into a continual cycle of monitoring and review that may, paradoxically, impede organic change and development". They propose the use of a critical paradigm which "understands that social work practice is uncertain, messy and complex (Fook, 2007) and which sees the role of evaluator as a critical friend (Balthasar, 2011) working alongside agencies and service users to co-create an evaluation that is owned by everyone (Whitmore, 2001). It becomes part-and-parcel of a self-reflexive, critical practice as described by Shaw and Shaw (1997), when they urged us to keep social work 'honest'".

We will now consider what Deliberate Practice can offer in response to these concerns, ethical dilemmas and paradoxes.

What Is Deliberate Practice and What Is It Not?

"Deliberate practice refers to a special type of practice that is purposeful and systematic. While regular practice might include mindless repetitions, deliberate practice requires focused attention and is conducted with the specific goal of improving performance" (Clear, 2016, p. 20). Deliberate Practice has been written about both in relation to habit change in everyday life (Clear, 2018) and in relation to expert performance (Ericsson, 2006).

Deliberate Practice has many interconnections with the Solution Focused approach, making it particularly useful for inclusion in Solution Focused coaching supervision. Some of what they share include:

- Both place learning from the clients at the centre, rather than privileging theory or other subject matter expert knowledge when it comes to maintaining and/or improving outcomes and effectiveness.
- Doing more of what already works is a simple but effective way to maintain practice that enables clients to accomplish the outcomes that they desire.

- Small changes can have significant effects. Hence iterative tweaks are favoured over complex changes. This allows what makes the difference that makes a valued difference, simple and clear to identify.
- Improvement requires that practitioners DO something different, not just talk about doing something different. This is particularly relevant for coaching supervision which can easily become a lot of talk that does not translate into capability improvements.
- Accountability and self-regulation are necessary for ethical practice. The way coaches go about their work, the methods they use and the activities they routinely engage with should prioritise and promote accountability and self-regulation.

In the remainder of this chapter these similarities between Deliberate Practice and the Solution Focused approach will become more evident as the details of Deliberate Practice and its implementation are described.

The Four Pillars of Deliberate Practice

Deliberate Practice is different from coaching practice. It consists of the following four building blocks, adapted to apply to coaching supervision (Miller et al., 2020):

1 A coaching supervisor who knows the coaching supervision client and can focus in on the details of their coaching, as well as zoom out to consider the bigger picture, namely their growth edge.
2 Individualised learning objectives – not just a general learning objective, but based on the baseline of the coaching supervision client's current practice.
3 Gathering performance feedback from clients in real time which is then used for learning from together with the coaching supervisor.
4 Generating progress through successive refinement by adopting an iterative process that takes place as the coaching supervision client's learning edge expands. This is not just repetition with the aim of practice making perfect, but rather with the aim of practice making permanent.

The aim is to create a cycle of excellence that is ongoing (Rousmaniere et al., 2017, p. 7), characterised by three components that are critical for superior performance (Miller et al., 2007):

- determining a baseline of effectiveness, including strengths and skills that need improvement,
- obtaining systematic ongoing formal feedback and
- engaging in Deliberate Practice.

Getting Started With Deliberate Practice

Effectiveness is all about doing the right thing, and doing it right. In order to become more effective, the coaching supervision client will need to know where they are in terms of effectiveness. Knowing their specific weaknesses can help them identify targets for their Deliberate Practice.

Firstly it is useful to identify what they are doing already that is working well – their Comfort Zone. Then the aim is to stretch out to their Learning Zone. This may be for example where their usual practice is less effective or falls short, where they are not helping certain clients in certain contexts or with certain issues as well as they usually do. The third zone is the Panic Zone where they are out of their depth, experience overwhelm or resistance, and are vulnerable to delivering poor practice. The first step in Deliberate Practice is therefore to get a baseline measure of their effectiveness.

Establishing a Baseline

There are two key areas to measure: overall effectiveness of the practice and the quality of the relationship (Miller et al., 2020). The two main measures that do this are the ORS (Miller & Duncan, 2000) and SRS (Miller et al., 2002), described below. These enable the coaching supervision client to rate how effective they are and how able they are to engage particular clients. They also allow the coaching supervision client to aggregate data over time in order to establish how effective they are overall, and where they may be less effective at engaging their coaching clients.

The Outcome Rating Scale (ORS)

The ORS (Miller & Duncan, 2000) provides a measure of a client's well-being in four different dimensions – individual, interpersonal, social and overall (see Figure 8.1). It is administered at the beginning of every coaching session. Clients' well-being is the overarching goal of psychotherapy. Coaching, however, is different as the goals coaching clients bring to a coaching process vary. The ORS would therefore need to be amended and individualised. A coach might ask their client about the main indicators for achieving what they want to achieve in the coaching process and create an individual ORS for each client, for example: "assertiveness, confidence, clear communication, overall" instead of "individual, interpersonal, social and overall".

These scales are being used by hundreds of thousands of practitioners around the world in diverse settings. They have been subjected to rigorous analysis and found to be both valid and reliable. They are also easy to use as they are brief and therefore possible to include in usual coaching appointments.

In order for the ORS to be useful, it is important to create a culture of feedback where the client is more likely to give forthright responses.

Outcome Rating Scale (ORS)

Name _____Age (Yrs):____ Gender_____
Session # ____ Date: _____
Who is filling out this form? Please check one: Self_____   Other_____
If other, what is your relationship to this person? _____

Looking back over the last week, including today, help us understand how you have been
feeling by rating how well you have been doing in the following areas of your life, where
marks to the left represent low levels and marks to the right indicate high levels. *If you are
filling out this form for another person, please fill out according to how you think he or she
is doing.*

Individually
(Personal well-being)

I--I

Interpersonally
(Family, close relationships)

I--I

Socially
(Work, school, friendships)

I--I

Overall
(General sense of well-being)

I--I

International Center for Clinical Excellence

www.centerforclinicalexcellence.com
www.scottdmiller.com

© 2000, Scott D. Miller and Barry L. Duncan

To obtain full working copies of these measures, please register online at:
http://www.scottdmiller.com/node/13

Figure 8.1 The outcome rating scale (ORS) (Miller & Duncan, 2000) (Reproduced
    with permission)

The instructions for introducing the ORS to clients are given below (Miller et al., 2020, p. 56, quoting Bargmann & Robinson, 2012, p. 9).

> My first priority is making sure that you get the results you want. For this reason, it is important that you are involved in monitoring progress. To do this, I used a brief measure called the Outcome Rating Scale. It takes about a minute to complete. I'll ask you to fill it out at the beginning of each session and then we'll talk about the results. A fair amount of research shows that if we are going to be successful in our work together, we should see signs of improvement sooner rather than later. If what we are doing works, then we'll continue. If not then we'll work together to figure out what we can do differently. If things still don't improve then we'll find someone or someplace else for you to get the help you want. Does this make sense to you?

Once the four scales have been personalised to the specific coaching client as outlined above, the client then makes a mark on the line that represents their current rating for the area they are working on and the coach measures the mark to the nearest millimetre. Adding the four lines together gives a total score of 40. This is then marked on the graph that is provided when you download the measure to track progress over time. Ideally the scores will go up over time. However, if the scores go down, this gives an opportunity to intervene early. If clients feel that they are not being helped, they may be less inclined to attend further sessions.

The Session Rating Scale (SRS)

The SRS (Miller et al., 2002) tells us the quality of the relationship from the client's point of view, often referred to as the working alliance. It is administered at the end of every session. There are four scales (see Figure 8.2) measuring:

- the quality of the relationship – feeling heard, understood and respected,
- goals and topics – working on what the client wanted to talk about,
- approach or method – is a good fit for the client and
- overall experience.

The original wording of the Approach or Method scale reads "therapist" and can easily be changed to "coach" once you have downloaded the tools from the link below.

Both the measures are available for use by individual practitioners at no cost as long as they register for a free licence here: http://scott-d-miller-ph-d. myshopify.com/collections/performance-metrics/products/performance-metrics-licenses-for-the-ors-and-srs

Session Rating Scale (SRS V.3.0)

Name ______________________Age (Yrs):____
ID# _______________________ Gender:_______
Session # ____ Date: ________________________

Please rate today's session by placing a mark on the line nearest to the description that best fits your experience.

Relationship

I did not feel heard, understood, and respected.	I--I	I felt heard, understood, and respected.

Goals and Topics

We did *not* work on or talk about what I wanted to work on and talk about.	I--I	We worked on and talked about what I wanted to work on and talk about.

Approach or Method

The therapist's approach is not a good fit for me.	I--I	The therapist's approach is a good fit for me.

Overall

There was something missing in the session today.	I--I	Overall, today's session was right for me.

International Center for Clinical Excellence

www.centerforclinicalexcellence.com
www.scottdmiller.com

To obtain full working copies of these measures, please register online at:
http://www.scottdmiller.com/node/13

Figure 8.2 The session rating scale (SRS) (Miller et al., 2002) (Reproduced with permission)

The SRS is introduced in the following way (Miller et al., 2020, p. 56, quoting Bargmann & Robinson, 2012, p. 14):

> I'd like to ask you to fill out one additional form. This is called the Session Rating Scale. A great deal of research shows that your experience of our work together – did you feel understood, did we focus on what

was important to you, did the approach I'm taking make sense and feel right – is a good predictor of whether we'll be successful. I want to emphasize that I'm not aiming for a perfect score – a 10 out of 10. Life isn't perfect and neither am I. What I'm aiming for is your feedback about even the smallest things – even if it seems unimportant – so we can adjust our work and make sure we don't steer off course. Whatever it might be, I promise I won't take it personally. I'm always learning and am curious about any feedback from you that will in time help me improve so I can better help you. Does that make sense?

Further Solution Focused questions (Dierolf et al., 2023) can be asked to get more detailed feedback from the coaching client either in relation to the four scales above or in relation to any other skill the coach has identified that they need to develop further in. Examples include:

- What were the instances when what we were doing together was just right for you?
- Where would you have wanted me to do this more?
- Where would you have wanted me to do this less?

"The main idea is to get client feedback, determine what you would like to work on, get more client feedback and work on it in preparation for the next session" (Dierolf et al., 2023, p. 192).

What to Do Once You Have a Baseline

Miller et al. (2020) provide an appendix in their book called the Taxonomy of Deliberate Practice Activities in Psychotherapy (TDPA). Appendix C (pp. 179–192) is the psychotherapy supervisor version and Appendix D is the therapist version (pp. 193–206).

This identifies five broad domains for Deliberate Practice, namely, structure, hope and expectancy, working alliance, client factors and practitioner factors. These were identified by Duncan et al. (2010) as factors accounting for the variability in outcomes.

Under each heading there are several questions for the coaching supervision client to ask of themselves and their own work, to rate their work in different areas and give details. The coaching supervisor rates the coaching supervision client according to the same areas. Both identify the top three areas that they believe would have a significant impact on improving the coaching supervision client's ability to engage with and support their clients' learning and growth. The ratings and top three activities to work on are then compared with the aim of coming to a consensus and using this as a platform for designing a clear learning objective to work on in coaching supervision – the stretch goal. This is then broken down into SMART (specific, measurable, attainable, relevant and time limited) goals, and a plan is made to have a routine of reviewing these.

Miller et al. (2017, pp. 37–38) recognise that sustaining Deliberate Practice can be challenging. They provide a clear structure to support Deliberate Practice using the acronym ARPS which stands for Automated structure, Reference point, Playful experimentation and Support. This is described below and can be shared with your coaching supervision clients.

1 Automated Structure

- Block out a specific regular weekly time for Deliberate Practice. One hour a week is recommended.
- Automate reminders for the time for Deliberate Practice.
- Set up a system to record all your sessions (after gaining client consent).

2 Reference Point

- Keep one eye on your outcome data (both individual and aggregated).
- Keep the other eye on your learning objectives.
- Take notes on a weekly basis to record learnings (they suggest noting the one thing that stands out that you want to remember).
- Choose a recording that represents you at your best, analyse what makes it stand out and take to your coaching supervisor for feedback.

3 Playful Experimentation

- Review a short segment of your recording (5–10 minutes) and consider how you might carry out the session more constructively.
- Seek to be surprised and disconfirmed by your client feedback – fill out the SRS at the same time as your client and compare the ratings to see what surprises you.

4 Support

- Find a coaching supervisor who is willing to listen to your recordings, incorporate data from the ORS and SRS into the discussions and help you develop key learning objectives rather than only discussing your coaching practice.

How to Use Deliberate Practice as a Coaching Supervisor

As coaching supervisors we can go through the process of Deliberate Practice for our own work both as a coach and as a coaching supervisor, as well as support our coaching supervision clients with their Deliberate Practice.

For our own work as a coach or coaching supervisor, we would need to establish what we do well (get our own baseline) and what our learning edge is. It may be wiser not to attempt to only self-supervise one's Deliberate Practice. Instead coaching supervisors can benefit from their own coaching supervision or ongoing work with a mentor coach.

Another way that you can use Deliberate Practice as a coaching supervisor is by helping your coaching supervision client focus on their own Deliberate Practice. It is very easy for coaching supervision to become a repetitive discussion of stuck cases that the supervision client brings. As noted earlier, accounts of what the coaching supervision client thinks about their effectiveness may not be aligned with what emerges when data on outcomes and effectiveness are gathered systematically and regularly. It is important to also watch recordings of sessions and have regular discussions about what the supervision client's overall learning goals are, informed by the feedback collected from the supervision client's clients, what they do well already and what the next noticeable steps would be that indicate they are making progress. Deliberate Practice is an ongoing interactive process, as once improvements are made, the next individualised learning goals are established and worked on and so on.

Providing Feedback

Ericsson (2006) recommends that feedback is incremental, split into chunks that are manageable by the learner, and is given in a way that does not elicit defensiveness that would affect the supervision client being able to hear and make use of the feedback. James (2015) suggests a seven step sequence for giving feedback:

1 Ensuring learners are aware of the purpose of the feedback.
2 Learners comment about the goals they were trying to achieve.
3 Learners state what features of the task they thought they had done well.
4 Supervisors state what features were done well.
5 Learners stating what could be improved.
6 Supervisor state what could be improved.
7 Together agree on action plans for improvement.

All this fits well with the Solution Focused approach to coaching supervision, which starts from a position of strengths, looks for next small steps forwards and aims to elicit ideas from the coaching supervision client and draws on their expertise before offering any ideas from the coaching supervisor's perspective.

Reflective Exercise: What Is Your Why?

After reading this chapter you may want to reflect on the following questions:

- Why do you want to be engaged in Deliberate Practice?
- What is important to you in your development as a coach and/or coaching supervisor?
- What motivates you and keeps you going?

- How can Deliberate Practice support you to become the kind of coach and/or coaching supervisor you wish to become?
- How would you like to support your coaching supervision clients by using Deliberate Practice to improve their outcomes and their effectiveness?

What Are Your Next Steps: Summary of Deliberate Practice

- Think about what you want to improve.
- Establish a baseline (SRS/ORS).
- Identify how you will know you are getting better.
- Watch real behaviour (video, audio, live).
- Get continuous, systematic feedback preferably from someone you like and trust and who supports your development goals, for example a coaching supervisor who makes use of Deliberate Practice.
- Develop and try out new ideas with a coaching supervisor.
- Establish a rhythm of practice, feedback and more practice.

Reflective Practice: A Companion of Deliberate Practice

The following chapter on Reflective Practice acts as a companion chapter to this chapter on Deliberate Practice. The most common definition of reflective practice in professional development comes from the work of Schön (1983) and is defined as "a dialogue of thinking and doing through which I become more skilful" (Schön, 1983, p. 56). Reflective Practice can be seen as a conversation focused on understanding, learning and figuring out what to take further from experiences and events, done over a period of time, with the purpose of expanding understanding and awareness. In this way Reflective Practice offers the coaching supervisor and the coaching supervision client a method to make sense of the data they gather during Deliberate Practice, as well as how to make well thought through selections of what to focus on in their improvement experiments and cycles of Deliberate Practice action implementation.

References

Balthasar, A. (2011). Critical friend approach: Policy evaluation between methodological soundness, practical relevance and transparency of the evaluation process. *German Policy Studies*, *7*(3), 187–231.

Chow, D. L., Miller, S. D., Seidel, J. A., Kane, R. T., Thornton, J. A., & Andrews, W. P. (2015). The role of deliberate practice in the development of highly effective psychotherapists. *Psychotherapy*, *52*(3), 337.

Clear, J. (2016) Deliberate practice guide. Retrieved from https://jamesclear.com/wp-content/uploads/2016/08/ABriefGuidetoDeliberatePractice.pdf?ref=blog.teambakery.com#:~:text=practicing%20and%20learning.-,JamesClear.com,something%20and%20passively%20learning%20it.%E2%80%9D

Clear, J. (2018). *Atomic habits*. Penguin Publishing Group.

Cree, V., Jain, S., & Hillen, P. (2018). Evaluating effectiveness in social work: Sharing dilemmas in practice. *European Journal of Social Work*, *22*, 1–12. https://doi.org/

10.1080/13691457.2018.1441136. Retrieved from https://www.researchgate. net/publication/323370072_Evaluating_effectiveness_in_social_work_sharing_ dilemmas_in_practice

Dierolf, K., Mühl, C., Perfetto, C., & Szaniawski, R. (2023). *Solution focused team coaching.* Taylor & Francis.

Duncan, B. L., Miller, S. D., Wampold, B. E., & Hubble, M. A. (2010). *The heart and soul of change: Delivering what works in therapy.* American Psychological Association.

Ericsson, K. A. (2006). The influence of experience and deliberate practice on the development of superior expert performance. In K.A. Ericsson, N. Charness, P.J. Feltovich & R.R. Hoffman (Eds.) *The Cambridge handbook of expertise and expert performance* (pp. 685–705). Cambridge University Press.

Fook, J. (2007). Uncertainty: The defining characteristic of social work? In M. Lymbery & K. Postle (Eds.) *Social work. A companion to learning.* Sage.

Goldberg, S. B., Rousmaniere, T., Miller, S. D., Whipple, J., Nielsen, S. L., Hoyt, W. T., & Wampold, B. E. (2016). Do psychotherapists improve with time and experience? A longitudinal analysis of outcomes in a clinical setting. *Journal of Counseling Psychology, 63*(1), 1–11. https://doi.org/10.1037/cou0000131

Hermel-Stanescu, M. (2015) *Effective coaching: key-factors that determine the effectiveness of a coaching program.* Bari, Italy. Management, Knowledge and Learning Joint International Conference. Retrieved from https://www.toknowpress.net/ ISBN/978-961-6914-13-0/papers/ML15-076.pdf

James, I. A. (2015). The rightful demise of the sh* t sandwich: Providing effective feedback. *Behavioural and Cognitive Psychotherapy, 43*(6), 759–766.

Miller, S. D., & Duncan, B. L. (2000). *The Outcome Rating Scale.* Author.

Miller, S. D., Duncan, B. L., & Johnson, L. D. (2002). *The Session Rating Scale 3.0.* Author.

Miller, S. D., Hubble, M. A., & Chow, D. (2017). Professional development: From oxymoron to reality. In T. Rousmaniere, R. K. Goodyear, S. D. Miller, & B. E. Wampold (Eds.), *The cycle of excellence: Using deliberate practice to improve supervision and training* (pp. 23–47).

Miller, S. D., Hubble, M. A., & Chow, D. (2020). *Better results: Using deliberate practice to improve therapeutic effectiveness.* American Psychological Association. https:// doi.org/10.1037/0000191-000

Miller, S. D., Hubble, M. A., & Duncan, B. L. (2007). Supershrinks: What's the secret of their success? *Psychotherapy Networker, 31*(6).

Rousmaniere, T., Goodyear, R., Miller, S. D., & Wampold, B. E. (2017). *The cycle of excellence: Using deliberate practice to improve supervision and training.* Wiley-Blackwell. https://doi.org/10.1002/9781119165590

Schön, D. A. (1983). *The reflective practitioner.* Basic Books.

Shaw, I., & Shaw, A. (1997). Keeping social work honest. Evaluating as profession and practice. *British Journal of Social Work, 27*(6), 847–869.

Whitmore, E. (2001). "People listened to what we had to say": Reflections on an emancipatory qualitative evaluation. In I. Shaw & N. Gould (Eds.) *Qualitative research in social work.* Sage.

9   The Role of Reflective Practice in Supervision

Cristina Mühl

Introduction to the Concept of Reflective Practice

The purpose of this chapter is to clarify what reflective practice is, how it can support the growth of any supervisor or coach and how it can be brought into the supervision space. As there are a multitude of models out there, the chapter starts with a short history and clarification of the term.

There are many definitions of the word "reflection" proposed by the Oxford Learner's Dictionaries (n.d.):

1   An image in a mirror, on a shiny surface, on water, etc.
2   The action or process of sending back light, heat, sound, etc. from a surface
3   A sign that shows the state or nature of something
4   Careful thought about something, sometimes over a long period of time
5   Your written or spoken thoughts about a particular subject or topic
6   An account or a description of something

As you might notice, all these definitions enhance the associations that we make with reflection and reflective practice in the coaching space. The act of reflecting implies writing or talking about something that needs careful thinking about and that will provide a mirror back.

The most common definition of reflective practice in professional development comes from the work of Schön (1983) and is defined as "a dialogue of thinking and doing through which I become more skilful" (Schön, 1983, p. 56). Reflective practice can be seen as a conversation focused on understanding, learning and figuring out what to take further from experiences and events, done over a period of time with the purpose of expanding understanding and awareness.

The concept of "reflective practice" seems to have appeared with Dewey (1896, p. 359) pointing out the distinction between the components of the "reflex arc" and making the point with an example of a child learning that the flame from a candle is hot – "child learn from the experience". From that incipient moment, several theories have been developed around reflection and reflective practice and its role in several professions: education, medicine,

DOI: 10.4324/9781003390527-9

engineering, leadership, coaching, supervision and so on. You can look at reflection as the activity and reflective practice as the way you engage with the process to create a continuous learning environment for yourself as a professional.

Reflective practice has vast applications and the way it has been used by diverse professions has shown that it can enhance the quality of the work of any practitioner. Before looking at the models in more detail, we will outline the link between reflective practice and both coaching and supervision competences.

The Link Between Reflective Practice and Coaching Competencies

The main coaching associations such as the International Coaching Federation (ICF), the European Mentoring and Coaching Council (EMCC) and Association for Coaching (AC) have developed competency models for individual coaching that have been in use for many years already. (ICF, n.d.; AC, 2012; EMCC, 2015). One of the areas where both ICF, AC and EMCC clearly overlap is the requirement for coaches to engage in reflection as part of their continuous development. ICF includes under Core competency number 2 – Embodies a Coaching Mindset the competency "Develops an ongoing reflective practice to enhance one's coaching" (ICF, n.d.). EMCC mentions "Demonstrates commitment to personal development through deliberate action and reflection" under the category Commitment to Self-Development in EMCC Competence Framework for individual coaching (EMCC, 2015). AC includes reflection in competency 9 "9. Undertaking continuous coach development" mentioning "Acts on own critical reflections and client feedback to improve coaching practice" as indicator of competence (AC, 2012).

Reflective practice also shows up also in the supervision competences and is seen as an important part of the EMCC Supervision Competence Framework (EMCC, 2019). Reflection is mentioned in:

- Competence 2 Facilitates Development: is where the supervisor "enables the supervisee to improve the standard of their practice through a process of facilitated reflection". This is further elaborated as competence 2.3 states "engages the supervisee in a process of critical reflection regarding their practice and supports them to develop their own reflective capability".
- Competence 5 Self-Awareness: the supervisor "develops their knowledge, understanding and awareness in relation to their self as a supervisor".

Making a case for reflective practice as a process focused on enhancing the skills, knowledge and quality offered in the coach's practice, understanding the different models and approaches would provide value as it would give insight into how it can be embedded in our coaching and supervision practice. Moreover, supervisors would be able to "engage the supervisee in a process of critical reflection regarding their practice and support them to develop their own reflective capability" in line with the EMCC Supervision Competence no. 2 Facilitates Development (EMCC, 2015). Gilbert and Trudel (2006, p. 113) suggest, "10 years of coaching without reflection is simply one year of coaching repeated 10 times".

Embedding Reflection in the Supervision Process

Some specific ways in which a coaching supervisor could bring reflection into the supervision work include:

1 Inviting the coaching supervision client to experiment with a guided reflection during a supervision session especially when the supervision client is bringing a case to supervision.
2 Dedicating space in a supervision session to have a conversation about quality in coaching and what can enhance it. Reflective practice is an important component in building quality evaluation in the coaching process.
3 Using reflection models in supervision conversations to model how reflection can be embedded in all conversations which encourage coaching supervision clients to bring it into their practice outside supervision and in their conversations with their clients.

Coaching supervision is a changing profession, currently building the body of knowledge that demonstrates the validity of the profession. Coaching supervisors are working at the edge of their knowledge to support coaching supervision clients, expand their practice and explore their professional identity. Building in a process of reflective practice ensures that coaching supervisors can respond to their coaching supervision clients in the moment and encourage their coaching supervision clients to do the same, while bringing self into the process by sharing their experience with reflective practice.

Coaching supervisors should also carry out their own process of reflective practice, to reflect and improve about their work as a coach as well as their work as a supervisor.

Introduction to Reflective Practice Models

There are several models that can be used to guide the reflection process and there is no single way of approaching it. We have selected some of the most commonly used models to provide a selection of potential applications, both from education and purposely developed for coaches.

We encourage the reader to select what fits their practice best and use what makes sense from each model with the aim of leading to enhanced awareness and development of their skills. The main models are outlined in Table 9.1 and then discussed in more detail.

Many of the models aim to use reflection as a way to extract meanings and understandings from a situation, to transform this into learning and next steps. As discussed in Chapter 3, the Solution Focused approach does not focus on

Table 9.1 Outline of Reflective Practice Models

Author and Focus	Main Steps
Borton (1970) – learning from the situation	1 What? 2 So what? 3 Now what?
Kolb (1984) – experiential learning	1 Concrete experience 2 Reflective observation 3 Abstract conceptualisation 4 Active experimentation
Gibbs (1988) – structured debriefing	1 Description 2 Feelings 3 Evaluation 4 Analysis 5 Conclusions 6 Action plan
Schön (1983) – value of knowledge from practice	1 Reflection in action 2 Reflection on action
Johns (2013) – moving from doing to being	1 Preparatory phase 2 Descriptive phase 3 Reflective phase – looking inwards 4 Anticipatory phase – looking outwards 5 Insight phase
Jackson (2004) – observing the reflective practice	1 Balance 2 Objectivity 3 Perspective 4 Capability
Hullinger et al. (2019) – integrated learning	1 Internal – Generalised 2 Internal – In-the-moment 3 External – Generalised 4 External – In-the-moment

diagnosing or uncovering "the truth" as we value pluralism, meaning we acknowledge there are multiple "truths". The supervisor aims at co-constructing the interaction and reflection.

After each model is outlined below, some Solution Focused questions are offered where appropriate that fit with each model. Later in the chapter, the development of a specific Solution Focused model of reflective practice (SOLUTION) is described with an illustrated example.

Learning From the Situation – Borton (1970)

Borton (1970) opened the exploration of reflective practice models by looking at how an educator or teacher could enhance the curriculum offered to

Model developed by: Borton (1970)
Focused on: Learning from the situation

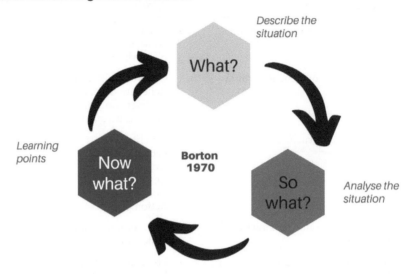

Figure 9.1 Reflective model developed by Borton (1970) (Image by Cristina Mühl)

students which could be transformative for their experience at school. He looked at students receiving a stimulus that was transformed into a result with three layers in between: sensing, transforming and acting. Those three layers were then conceptualised to What?, So what? Now what? (see Figure 9.1).

The very simplistic structure of the model makes it very accessible and easy to implement in any conversation structure. Borton mentions:

> The what, so what, now what sequence should be a continuous integrated flow. Do not expect students to begin at some 'beginning' and end at some 'end', for beginning at any point should lead back through the same sequence. Start where the students are, and pick up the other parts of the process as they seem appropriate. If the sequence no longer seems helpful in a real situation, then abandon theory and follow intuition. ... when the model does not prove useful, change it.
>
> (Borton, 1970, p. 94)

Solution Focused questions that can be implemented:

- For the "So what?" step
  - "What would you like instead of that?"
  - "What would have been your best hopes about that situation that you are describing?"

- For the "Now what?" step

  - "What would be the smallest step that you can take in the next 24 hours that will allow you to learn something from this situation?"
  - "What would you notice once you approach the situation differently next time?" "What would others notice?"

Experiential Learning – Kolb (1984)

Experiential learning is defined by Kolb (1984, p. 20) "to emphasise the central role that experience plays in the learning process".

His desire was not to offer one more model that should be placed above other learning theories such as behavioural (focus on observable behaviours and the way the environment influences behaviour) or cognitive (focus on the role of mental processes in learning), but wanted to suggest a holistic perspective. The model makes the case that "learning is the process whereby knowledge is created through the transformation of experience" (Kolb, 1984, p. 38). It encompasses the belief that "knowledge is a transformation process, being continuously created and recreated, not an independent entity to be acquired or transmitted" (Kolb, 1984, p. 38). Hence, learning is the process of creating knowledge.

The model starts from a concrete experience. Practitioners need to be able to "fully, openly and without bias" (Kolb, 1984, p. 30) involve themselves in the concrete experience, reflect upon it, conceptualise the experience and then engage again in active experimentation. As you might notice the activities are opposed and that was intentional in the view of Kolb (1984).

> There are two primary dimensions to the learning process. The first dimension represents the concrete experience of events at one end and abstract conceptualization at the other. The other dimension has active experimentation at one extreme and reflective observation at the other. Thus, in the process of learning, one moves in varying degrees from actor to observer, and from specific involvement to general analytic detachment.
>
> (Kolb, 1984, pp. 30–31)

Figure 9.2 summarises these dimensions.
Solution Focused questions that can be used with the model include:

- Abstract conceptualisation

  - "What name would you give to this situation?"
  - "What would be something that will remind you of it?"

- Active experimentation

  - "What is the smallest step you could try?"
  - "What do you want to experiment with in a similar situation?"

Model developed by: Kolb (1984)
Focuses on: Experiential learning

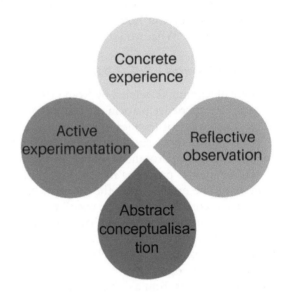

Figure 9.2 Reflective model developed by Kolb (1984) (Image by Cristina Mühl)

Structured Debriefing – Gibbs (1988)

Basing his thoughts on the model developed by Kolb (1984), Gibbs (1988) aimed at bringing examples of how learning can be enhanced by doing. While presenting different tools for exploring what Kolb called "reviewing", Gibbs introduced the term "structured debriefing". The model remains highly relevant for turning practice into theory – "The suggestion is therefore that learners ought to be using practice in order to develop and test theory and not the other way round" (Gibbs, 1988, p. 8).

Methods described by Gibbs are designed to provide any teacher a summary of tools and ideas that can support "experiential learning". He considers that "it is not sufficient simply to have an experience in order to learn. Without reflecting upon this experience it may quickly be forgotten or its learning potential lost" (Gibbs, 1988, p. 14). This is one of the key roles that coaching supervision plays, to support the coaching supervision client in making its sense of the experience and co-creating a future where those learnings are put to use.

The reflective cycle proposed by Gibbs (1988) includes the following six stages which are then shown in Figure 9.3:

- Description (What happened? What was the event all about?)
- Feelings (What were you feeling? What were you thinking?)

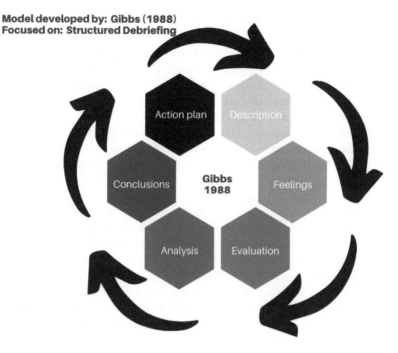

Figure 9.3 Reflective model developed by Gibbs (1988) (Image by Cristina Mühl)

- Evaluation (Was the experience good or bad?)
- Analysis (What can you understand from the situation?)
- Conclusion (What else could you have done?)
- Action plan (What do you want to do if you are faced with a similar situation?)

From a Solution Focused stance, there is a need to clarify whether looking at the levels of "Feelings", "Evaluation" and "Analysis" is needed.

The Reflective Practitioner – Schön (1983)

The work done by Schön (1983) to raise the awareness of the knowledge that practitioners bring in each field and how that should be seen as at least as valuable as the expertise brought by researchers, had a great impact on the transformation of the professional body of knowledge and balancing the scale between the researchers and practitioners. In his first book, Schön (1983) made the case that professions should not be classified based on the level of academic work and that they should not be seen as below the academic world. There is plenty of knowledge embedded in practitioners.

In "The Reflective Practitioner", Schön mentions

> as one would expect from the hierarchical model of professional knowledge, research is institutionally separate from practice, connected to it by carefully defined relationships of exchange. Researchers are supposed to provide the basic and applied science from which to derive techniques for diagnosing and solving the problems of practice. Practitioners are supposed to furnish researchers with problems for study and with tests of the utility of research results. The researcher's role is distinct from, and usually considered superior to, the role of the practitioner.
>
> (Schön, 1983, p. 26)

Based on the assumption that practitioners bring highly valuable input and that there are elements in their practice done by intuition, Schön (1983) offered a reflective model constructed around the moment when the reflection takes place: "in action", meaning while things are happening and "on action" after the event/interaction took place already (see Figure 9.4).

This is the aim of reflective practice, e.g. that by consciously reflecting after the event regularly it means it will be easier to reflect while in the session with a client so that you can move from being reflective to reflexive.

Model developed by: Schön (1983)
Focused on: The value of knowledge from practice

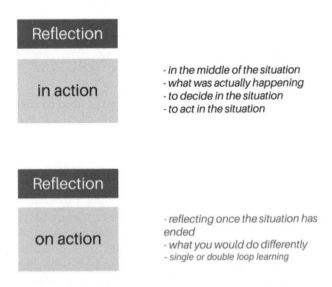

Figure 9.4 Reflective model developed by Schön (1983) (Image by Cristina Mühl)

Being reflective means actively thinking about an event after it happened and exploring it with the desire to learn from it and obtain insights. Being reflexive implies that we are actively taking our surroundings into account and critically reflecting in the moment on the events and acting based on our enhanced understanding.

Some Solution Focused questions that can be used for "Reflection in action":

- "If this action/conversation turns out to be useful, what needs to happen?"
- "What are my best hopes for this situation?"
- "What would I notice that would tell me that this situation turned out right?"

From Doing to Being Reflective – Johns (2013)

Johns highlights that "reflective practices span from doing reflection towards being reflective. Doing reflection reflects an epistemological approach, as if reflection is a tool or device. Indeed, this is true to an extent. However, reflection is much more than that. Being reflective reflects an ontological approach. It is about 'who I am' rather than 'what I do'" (Johns, 2013, Chapter 1, "Reflection on experience", para 1).

A particularly interesting aspect brought by Johns is the link to empowerment. "Empowerment is the practitioner having the commitment and courage to take action towards realising more effective practice and a better state of affairs" (Johns, 2013, Chapter 1, "Empowerment", para 4). This view on reflective practice is in line with the role of coaching supervision, to create a space where the coaching supervision client is empowered to take ownership of their further development and co-create the path forward.

Besides constructing a framework of how to analyse the situation and observe patterns of knowing, Johns (2013) also proposed a model of structured reflection (MSR). These stages are described below and illustrated in Figure 9.5:

- Preparatory phase ("bring the mind home" involves mindfulness and creating a space for ourselves)
- Descriptive phase (describe the experience with both positive and negative sides)
- Reflective phase (reflection on several layers such as one's feelings, feelings of others, responses, intent of actions and reactions, prior experience, assumptions that govern practice, etc.)
- Anticipatory phase (reframing the situation to respond differently, and what are the consequences on others, factors constraining the response)
- Insight phase (what emerged)

Model developed by: Johns (2013)
Focused on: Moving from doing to being

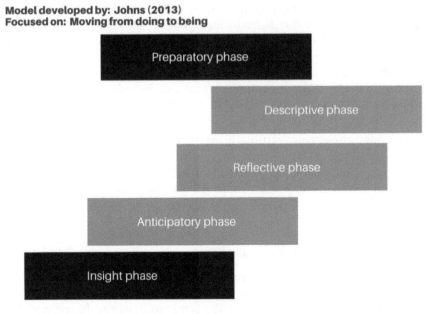

Figure 9.5 Reflective model developed by Johns (2013) (Image by Cristina Mühl)

Solution Focused questions that can be used in the different phases of the model include:

- Reflective phase
    - "What do you notice?"
    - "What have others noticed?"
- Anticipatory phase
    - "What would you like instead of that?"
    - "What difference would that make to you?"
- Insight phase
    - "What becomes now possible?"
    - "What emerges for you?"

The models presented above have wide applications across many professions. While none were explicitly designed with coaching in mind, they can still be helpful to coaching supervisors to use with coaching supervision clients either through guided reflection in a coaching supervision session or supporting the coaching supervision client to use outside the session in the process of reflecting on their coaching practice. There have however in recent years been models developed specifically with coaching in mind. These are discussed below.

Models of Reflective Practice in Coaching

A Four-Cornered Model of the Mechanism of Reflection in Coaching – Jackson (2004)

Jackson (2004) started by looking at reflective practice as a general concept, drawing parallels to coaching practice and how based on observed reflections, by simply asking the question "Why did this help?", a new structure of reflective practice emerged focused on coaching practice.

A very practical model emerged that allows coaches to reflect using a structure that

> brings two essential functions together. It provides a method of understanding that is sufficiently linked to both theory and to the reality of practice. Reflection works because it helps the learner to Balance the process of learning from experience and to generate new learning opportunities; it affords them an Objective stance; it helps them see their actions from the Perspective of their overall goals; and it helps them to develop the Capability to react more quickly and effectively to future challenges. These benefits are demonstrable in a coaching context and may provide an understanding of the importance of reflection to support and guide coaching practice.
>
> (Jackson, 2004, p. 66)

The steps of the model are outlined in Figure 9.6.

Balance refers to stimulating and discovering learning processes, especially the ones that are not the "preferred styles" (Jackson, 2004, p. 62) and activating those to enrich the reflection. Objectivity implies that after the event we can look at it after the emotions have passed and we can view the experience objectively. Perspective stage requires to look at the experience and pose the question "what do you really want?", hence allowing for the wider goal in mind. Capability turns the reflection into a habit and allows for reflection in action.

Some examples of Solution Focused question that can be used in "Balance":

- "What has been useful for you in other learning situations?"
- "How do you explore best past experiences?"

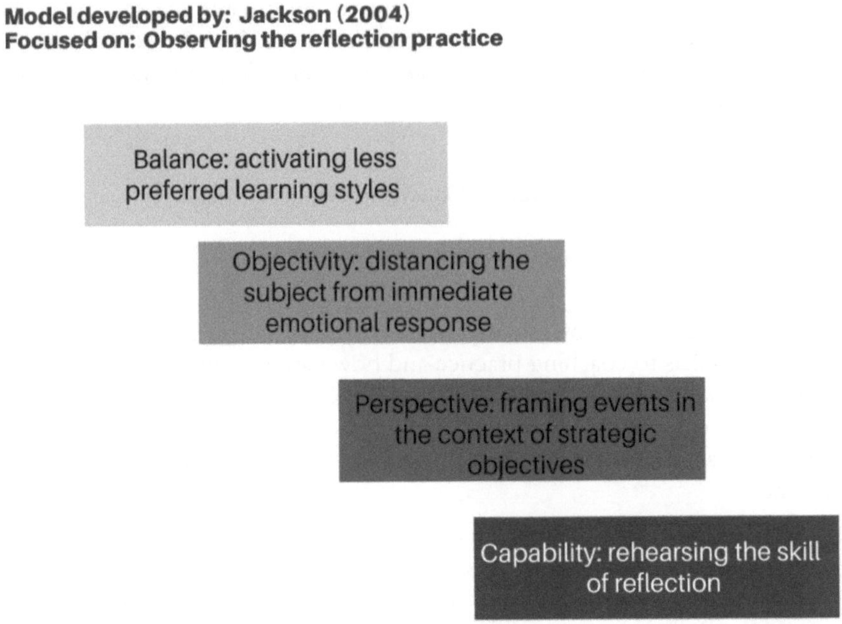

Model developed by: Jackson (2004)
Focused on: Observing the reflection practice

Balance: activating less preferred learning styles

Objectivity: distancing the subject from immediate emotional response

Perspective: framing events in the context of strategic objectives

Capability: rehearsing the skill of reflection

Figure 9.6 Reflective model developed by Jackson (2004) (Image by Cristina Mühl)

An Integrated Model for Learning – Hullinger et al. (2019)

One of the first steps taken towards creating a model that has the coaching profession in mind was done by Hullinger and colleagues in 2019, the graphic summary is Cristina's (Figure 9.7). Their model aims at bringing together three key concepts from coaching: reflection, awareness and self-regulation. All three concepts are related to "one's past or present experiences to examine one's own character, thoughts, behaviour, emotions, beliefs, motivations, and abilities and how others perceive the person". Reflection means to contemplate, observe, inspect and question without judgement. "Awareness is defined as a clear, accurate perception and appraisal of those elements and self-regulation means to exercise control of or to modify one's present or future emotions and behaviour in order to act in accordance with the situation and the person's desired goals and plan" (Hullinger et al., 2019, p. 19). It's structured in two dimensions: Internal – External and Generalised – In-the-Moment.

Hullinger et al. mention

reflection is an engagement process for observing and questioning. Reflection evokes awareness; awareness activates self-regulation. Once self-regulation has occurred, a person can return to reflection by

Model developed by: Hullinger, DiGirolamo, Tkach (2019)
Focused on: Integrated learning

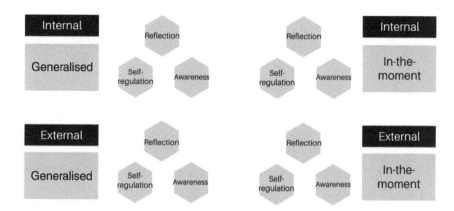

Figure 9.7 Reflective model developed by Hullinger et al. (2019) (Image by Cristina Mühl)

observing and questioning the changes in behaviour or emotion and new experience. The interactive process for reflecting, gaining awareness, and self-regulating is a learning experience that facilitates change.

(Hullinger et al., 2019, p. 20)

As a process the coach is invited to reflect after each session on the feelings, emotions, thoughts, triggers, etc. that came up during the coaching session (see Figure 9.8). This allows for awareness to be created that leads to generating a plan to self-regulate. The same flow from reflection, awareness and self-regulation would be followed also in the moment. The authors encouraged applying the same flow also in the coaching sessions, by offering coaching clients questions that mirror the reflection, awareness and self-regulation steps.

As the model was developed to enhance the flow between reflection, awareness and self-regulation, that same flow can be embedded in a coaching supervision session. The supervision client can be guided through those steps to look at different situations from their coaching practice.

Some Solution Focused questions that can be used include:

- "What story tells you that?"
- "What are you becoming aware of?"
- "What steps do you want to take next time?"

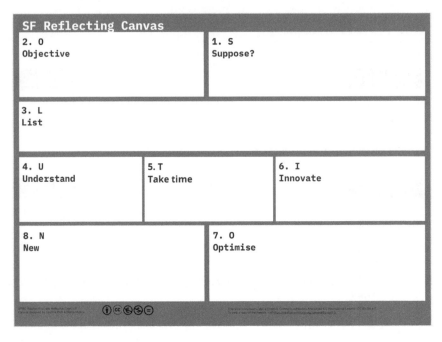

Figure 9.8 Reflective model developed by Mühl and Matera (2021) (Image by Cristina Mühl)

A Solution Focused Approach to Reflective Practice – SOLUTION

The desire to explore what a specific Solution Focused reflection would look like started from peer conversations between Cristina Mühl and Marco Matera. Both embarked on constructing a process that would encompass the Solution Focused tenets and serve as a model that allows self-reflection and guided reflection with a coaching supervisor.

SOLUTION (Mühl & Matera, 2021) came to life as a flexible structure that can be embedded within the calendar of any practitioner as it's based on the assumptions that reflection happens all the time and that the future is co-created through the interactions.

It involves a series of steps that can be adjusted to fit the purpose of the reflection using the acronym SOLUTION. Each of the steps with useful questions is outlined in Table 9.2. The answers to the questions can be summarised on the SOLUTION canvas (Figure 9.8) shown below the table.

As you might notice, the model incorporates several of the Solution Focused tenets and moves (more on Solution Focused supervision moves can be found in Chapter 3). It creates a playful space to explore either a case or a general topic.

Table 9.2 Steps in the SOLUTION Model (Mühl & Matera, 2021)

SOLUTION	
S – **Suppose**	• Suppose this reflective practice/supervision turns out to be useful for you, what might be different?
O – **Objective/s**	• And what difference might that make? • What might become possible then? • What are the benefits?
L – **List**	• What are all the things that are relevant to consider during your reflection? • For example, all the things that went well; all the things where there were opportunities you did not take, all the things you chose not to pick up on/ respond to in the client's contributions.
U – **Understanding**	• What are you becoming aware of in relation to this client / piece of coaching? • With the data from the list/s, what possibilities emerge about how to do things differently?
T – **Take time**	• What are the early/obvious conclusions you could jump too? • What else might you conclude/learn? And where can that take you? • What can you acknowledge and appreciate about yourself as a coach in this piece of coaching with this client? • And … take time. Go for a walk, engage with something else, allow for the thinking to take place.
I – **Innovate**	• How might you put this into action? What might you be doing and being if you went beyond the obvious/ your usual practice?
O – **Optimise**	• How confident are you now at being able to coach with this client? • What can you draw on to support you in your future coaching?
N – **Now/new**	• What is the smallest, simplest thing that you can implement/experiment with that you'd like to give a go?

When we look at the landscape of in-action vs on-action, the model allows for a thorough reflection on-action post event. Once the practitioner becomes familiar with the steps, they could experiment with using a shorter version of the model in the moment and look at LUI – List, Understand, Innovate. That allows for small incremental experiments that can provide valuable insights in a conversation.

Reflective Practice Example Using the SOLUTION Model

The following reflection is documented following a coaching session with a client seeking to understand how to position himself for a promotion.

S – Suppose	• Suppose this reflective practice/supervision turns out to be useful for you, what might be different? *To make best use of this reflection time I would need to come to a different way of approaching clients that come in with career coaching topics.*
O – Objective/s	• And what difference might that make? • What might become possible then? • What benefits? *I guess the main difference for me would be to simply feel that I'm sitting entirely in the coach seat and not moving into any advice giving or feeling too empathetic towards the client as the career development process is not easy.* *And if I will be able to do that, then I will be serving the client more and trusting them that they can find their way. For the client probably more empowerment that they will sort it out and for me – I will be closing the session feeling uplifted and not with a question mark.*
L – List	• What are all the things that are relevant to consider during your reflection? For example, all the things that went well; all the things where there were opportunities you did not take? All the things you chose not to pick up on/respond to in the client's contributions. *This particular session that generated the reflection was with a client that was feeling overstepped in the promotion and recognition of the work done. He was asked to step in and take responsibility for quite challenging projects informally and formally, he was still in the organisational structure at a junior level. He was now looking into an internal application for a promotion. That would have been about the level that he was informally.* *What went well in the session was that I would support the client to become aware of all the resources that helped him get also the informal moves in the company. He was able to reflect and match his own values with the company ones and to what the job required.* *There was a moment when he realised that what he needs is advice on getting his application ready. And that was the moment that was challenging. I could see that he had no prior experience in presenting himself, as all projects were offered based on prior results and by managers that trusted him.*

(*Continued*)

That resonated with me as it was a familiar feeling from the start of my career when I was in a similar state: doing the projects without formal recognition. The director of the department was aware that I can handle any project, but I was not formally given the job.

U – Understanding
- What are you becoming aware of in relation to this client/piece of coaching?
- With the data from the list/s what possibilities emerge about how to do things differently?

I think that one element that emerges is that we as coaches, of course we are part of the conversation. We bring ourselves to the session and there will be moments when we are not completely present to attend to the client. I guess what is more important is how we notice that and get back on track. Even how do we partner with the client to bring that to the conversation and see what is useful from that moment.

And I guess that is what makes us human and human coaching, different from engaging with an AI coach.

Possibilities that emerge from this are around partnering with the client from the contracting phase; knowing that this is normal and it's not a coach failure I think helps; talking to peers to see how they work with similar situations.

T – Take time
- What are the early/obvious conclusions you could jump too?
- What else might you conclude/learn? And where can that take you?
- What can you acknowledge and appreciate about yourself as coach in this piece of coaching with this client?
- And … take time. Go for a walk, engage with something else, allow for the thinking to take place.

Returning from a walk in the forest I realise that the time taken was useful to come to terms with the situation and with the fact that it will happen a lot to have clients that might have a career path or something that will resonate with me.

That is fine, it's not showing that I've missed something in my developmental process or that I have not committed strong enough to competencies and standards. It's just a human interaction and that is not free of co-creation.

I – Innovate
- How might you put action into action? What might you be doing and being if you went beyond the obvious/your usual?

Besides the ideas above and the usual to go talk to my supervisor or peers, there is another idea the comes up -> I would be curious to see if there has been any research or exploration done around the way the definition of coaching influences the way we approach it or the coach.

(*Continued*)

O – Optimise	• How confident are you now at being able to coach with this client? • What can you draw on to support you in your future coaching? *My confidence level increased after the walk. It was useful to take the break and not feel like I'm pressured to come up with an idea and stick to it. With this particular client, I'll go ahead and take at the start of our next session some time to recontract.* *The ideas generated through the reflection will certainly help with coming out of the session with that feeling of this was a good session and I haven't been stepping out of the coaching framework.*
N – Now/new	• What is the smallest, simplest thing that you can implement/experiment with that you'd like to give a go? *The smallest step that I can take is to dedicate 30 minutes to a short review of the session notes and see what I can take in the next conversation to support the recontracting with the client.*

Reflective Exercise

• What do you already do to reflect on your practice (e.g. when do you do it, how do you do it, what do you reflect on?)
• What works well from your existing reflective practice that you want to keep going forwards?
• From reading this chapter, what small steps are you inspired to try that might improve your reflective practice even more?
• As a coaching supervisor, how will you use these ideas to build the process of reflective practice with your coaching supervision clients?

References

Association for Coaching (2012). *AC coaching competency framework.* Retrieved from https://cdn.ymaws.com/www.associationforcoaching.com/resource/resmgr/Accreditation/Accred_General/Coaching_Competency_Framewor.pdf
Borton, T. (1970). *Reach, touch, and teach.* McGraw-Hill.
Dewey, J. (1896). The reflex arc concept in psychology. *Psychological Review, 3*(4), 359.
European Mentoring and Coaching Council (2015). *EMCC Global Competences Framework V2.* Retrieved from https://www.emccglobal.org/leadership-development/competences/
European Mentoring and Coaching Council (2019). EMCC Global Supervision Competence Framework. Retrieved from https://www.emccglobal.org/wp-content/uploads/2022/01/EMCC-competences-supervision-EN.pdf
Gibbs, G. (1988). *Learning by doing: A guide to teaching and learning methods.* Further Education Unit at Oxford Polytechnic.

Gilbert, W., & Trudel, P. (2006) The coach as a reflective practitioner. In Jones, R. L. (ed.) *The sports coach as educator: Reconceptualising sports coaching.* Routledge, pp. 113–127

Hullinger, A. M., DiGirolamo, J. A., & Tkach, J. T. (2019). Reflective practice for coaches and clients: An integrated model for learning. *Philosophy of Coaching: An International Journal, 4*(2), 5–34.

International Coaching Federation (n.d.). *Core competencies.* Retrieved February 9, 2024, from https://coachingfederation.org/credentials-and-standards/core-competencies

Jackson, P. (2004). Understanding the experience of experience: A practical model of reflective practice for coaching. *International Journal of Evidence Based Coaching and Mentoring, 2*(1), 57.

Johns, C. (2013). *Becoming a reflective practitioner (4th Ed).* Wiley-Blackwell.

Kolb, D. A. (1984). *Experiential learning, experience as the source of learning and development.* Prentice-Hall.

Mühl, C., & Matera, M. (2021). SOLUTION for your reflective practice. *European Mentoring and Coaching Council Romania.* Online. April 13, 2021.

Oxford Learner's Dictionaries (n.d.). Reflection. Retrieved February 3, 2024, from https://www.oxfordlearnersdictionaries.com/definition/english/reflection?q=reflection

Schön, D. A. (1983). *The reflective practitioner.* Basic Books.

10 Mentor Coaching

Svea van der Hoorn, Carlo Perfetto and Chris Bekker

Introduction

Words create worlds, and words evoke meanings which can create shared understandings or misunderstandings. These can support or disturb interpersonal relationships and communications. This chapter is devoted to International Coaching Federation (ICF) mentor coaching, as distinguished from other uses of the word mentor and mentoring. Mentoring and mentor coaching are located as overlapping with coaching supervision in purpose and function. Mentoring describes the relationship between a person with more expertise and experience who supports the aspirations of someone in their career development. Mention is made of the European Mentoring and Coaching Council's (EMCC's) stance on mentoring.

ICF mentor coaching is located as a subset of coaching supervision. It has a very specific purpose and set of requirements that must be complied with. ICF mentor coaching forms part of the ICF gold standard quality framework. The role, competencies, duties and responsibilities of a mentor coach are outlined. Mentor coaching focuses on the ongoing development of a coach's ability to demonstrate the ICF core competencies in their coaching.

The chapter foregrounds a vital function of coaching supervision and ICF mentor coaching, namely, the generating and giving of feedback – both written and verbal. Attention is paid to the complex task that ICF mentor coaches face in providing feedback that is both quality assurance informed and focused on the development of coaching capability. This includes the management of bias and/or blindspots. Extracts from a transcript are offered to illustrate ICF mentor coaching in action.

The terms "mentoring" and "mentor" are not exclusive to the world of mentor coaching, nor to the world of coaching supervision. We invite the reader to reflect on their current understanding/s of the terms "mentor", "mentoring" and "mentor coaching" and to refresh, revise and/or expand how they would talk with a coach about what they include in their service offerings. What they offer may be part of coaching supervision or a separate service.

For clarity purposes, we are delimiting the term "ICF mentor coaching" to the activity that is part of the ICF quality framework for Coach Education

DOI: 10.4324/9781003390527-10

(ICF CE) and Credentialing and Standards (ICF C&S). "Mentor Coaching for an ICF credential consists of coaching and feedback in a collaborative, appreciative and dialogued process based on an observed or recorded coaching session to increase the coach's capability in coaching, in alignment with the ICF Core Competencies" (International Coaching Federation, n.d. a).

We are also offering a short overview of mentoring in the EMCC framework to highlight where the practices might overlap and where they differ according to the ICF and EMCC frameworks (EMCC Global, n.d.).

The Purpose, Function and Demarcations of Mentoring and Mentor Coaching in the Coaching Community

In the coaching community confusion arises due to the same word being used to refer to different services and/or activities. Some coaches seek mentoring from a coach who they consider has more expertise, and who is willing and able to guide them in developing their career and their confidence as a professional coach. Some coaches are focused on achieving career development by successfully applying for certification with a professional coaching organisation like ICF or EMCC. To add to the confusion, each professional organisation has its own requirements and its own terminology to describe these. Some coaches seek coaching supervision hoping to have access to more comprehensive career development support that includes support and guidance about the technical aspects of coaching, for example, coaching competencies, support and guidance in trouble-shooting difficulties experienced in their coaching practice with clients, and support and guidance in maintaining their well-being in the face of the demands of working in the area of people development and growth. Some coaches seek coaching supervision as a compliance exercise – to meet the requirements of a professional coaching organisation, an employer of internal coaches, contractors of external coaches and/or individual buyers of coaching. Let's reflect on how mentoring is similar to and different from ICF mentor coaching.

Mentoring and ICF mentor coaching are related concepts, but they serve somewhat different purposes. Let's explore some similarities and differences.

Similarities Between Mentoring and ICF Mentor Coaching

Relationship focus: Both mentoring and ICF mentor coaching involve a supportive relationship between an experienced coach (mentor or mentor coach) and a less experienced coach (mentee or mentor coaching client).

Professional development: Both aim to contribute to the development of the coach. This development may encompass expanding and/or strengthening coaching skills, developing ethical maturity and decision-making and/or overall competency in relation to the quality standards of the coaching profession.

Ethical coaching practice: Both seek to promote ethical coaching practice and hence the coach's ability and commitment to do good, not harm. Mentoring does this by offering examples from the mentor's experience that are relevant to the mentee's development and situation. The ICF mentor coach does this by exploring with the coach how to demonstrate core competency 1: *Demonstrates ethical coaching practice*, and CC2: *Embodies a coaching mindset*, in their coaching.

Differences Between Mentoring and ICF Mentor Coaching

Purpose: The primary purpose of mentoring is to provide support, guidance and advice based on the mentor's own experiences and expertise. Mentoring often covers a broader range of topics beyond coaching skills, including career development, work-life balance, business development and personal growth. On the other hand, ICF mentor coaching is specifically focused on enhancing coaching skills and competencies to meet ICF credentialing requirements. The goal is for the coach to develop and refine their coaching abilities in alignment with ICF core competencies, at the level of credential that they are applying for (International Coaching Federation, n.d. a).

ICF credentialing: While mentoring may contribute to a coach's overall professional development, it does not necessarily fulfil the specific requirements for ICF credentialing. The mentoring process might not explicitly address the criteria set by the ICF for obtaining credentials. The ICF mandates a specific number of mentor coaching hours must be undertaken to meet credential requirements. ICF mentor coaching sessions must focus on coaching skills development, and the ICF mentor coach needs to comply with specific ICF criteria.

Competency development: In a mentoring relationship, the mentor draws upon their experience to guide the mentoring client in various aspects of their personal and professional development. The emphasis may not be solely on coaching competencies/standards. By contrast, the focus of ICF mentor coaching is on enhancing and fine-tuning the coach's demonstration of ICF core competencies. It involves providing feedback on live or recorded coaching sessions so that the coach can develop their coaching capability to make the core competencies discernible in their coaching, no matter what coaching model/approach they draw on and no matter what their coaching style.

In summary, while both mentoring and ICF mentor coaching involve a supportive relationship aimed at professional development, ICF mentor coaching is more narrowly focused on developing coaching skills and competencies according to specific ICF criteria.

The ICF Perspective on Mentor Coaching

The primary purpose of ICF mentor coaching is to assist coaches to meet the requirements set for obtaining or renewing ICF credentials. During ICF mentor coaching, the mentor coach guides the mentor coaching client to apply and demonstrate the ICF core competencies effectively in their coaching practice. This involves criteria-referenced assessment, providing feedback and support to ensure that the requirements are met. It includes reflective discussions and deliberate practice activities to help the coach deepen their understanding and application of the ICF core competencies.

Many coaches find ICF mentor coaching to be a desirable form of continuous improvement beyond securing or renewing an ICF credential. ICF mentor coaching for ongoing development aims to enhance the coach's proficiency in consistently applying the ICF core competencies in a variety of coaching contexts and with a variety of coaching clients. Coaches may engage in mentor coaching throughout their career to refine their skills and stay aligned with evolving coaching standards. It is particularly useful for coaches who wish to expand their existing coaching capability in relation to different socio-cultural norms and ways of living that come with expanding services into new markets. Thus they increase their coaching capacity to be attuned to the diversity of their coaching clients. As their coaching practices evolves, ongoing ICF mentor coaching helps coaches stay current, be flexible and adaptable, and hence future fit.

ICF mentor coaching encourages a commitment to professional growth and ensures that coaches remain effective and competent in their coaching engagements by delivering on the promise to buyers of coaching who specifically select an ICF credential holder.

The EMCC Perspective on Mentor Coaching

The EMCC recognises the term "mentor coaching" as a distinct concept from mentoring within their competency framework. EMCC defines mentor coaching and how it differs from mentoring as follows:

	EMCC Mentor Coaching	*EMCC Mentoring*
Purpose	Mentor coaching is specifically focused on developing the coaching skills and competence of individuals who are already coaches or aspire to become coaches	Mentoring is a broader concept aimed at supporting the personal and professional development of an individual, referred to as the mentee
Target audience	Mentor coaching is typically targeted at individuals who are engaged in or seeking to enter the coaching profession	Mentoring can extend to various fields, including coaching, leadership, career development and more. It is not exclusively focused on individuals within the coaching profession
Focus	The primary focus of mentor coaching is on enhancing the coach's coaching skills, methodologies and overall professional competence	While mentoring may involve discussions about coaching skills, it encompasses a wider range of topics related to the mentee's overall growth, career advancement and personal development

(Continued)

	EMCC Mentor Coaching	*EMCC Mentoring*
Process	Mentor coaching involves a collaborative and reflective process where the mentor coach works with the individual to deepen their understanding of coaching principles, improve their coaching techniques and enhance their ability to facilitate the growth and development of their coaching clients	Mentoring involves a supportive and guidance-oriented relationship where the mentor shares their knowledge, experiences and insights to help the mentee navigate challenges, set goals and achieve desired outcomes

In summary, EMCC mentor coaching is seen as a specialised form of support tailored for individuals involved in or aspiring to enter the coaching profession. This is different from the ICF perspective where mentor coaching is a requirement for seasoned coaches with 100–2500+ client coaching hours) to be awarded post-entry level coaching credentials. It concentrates on refining coaching skills and competencies. In contrast, mentoring is a broader relationship that focuses on the overall development of the mentee, covering various aspects beyond coaching skills and applicable to a wider range of professional and personal contexts (Lucas, 2020). The purpose of mentor coaching is something ICF and EMCC share. However, for ICF coaches engaging in mentor coaching is mandatory to ensure compliance with the ICF quality assurance framework.

Characteristics, Duties and Responsibilities of ICF Mentor Coaches, EMCC Mentor Coaches and Coaching Supervisors

The ICF has established clear standards outlining the characteristics, duties and responsibilities of ICF mentor coaches (International Coaching Federation, n.d. a). EMCC has done the same for coaching supervisors (EMCC Global, 2019). Whereas ICF mentor coaches are expected to be equipped to undertake criteria-referenced assessments to generate their feedback, EMCC mentor coaches and coaching supervisors need to be skilled in facilitating reflective practice.

ICF Mentor Coach and EMCC Coach Supervisor Characteristics and Capabilities

ICF

Ethical conduct: The adherence to a strong ethical framework, ensuring integrity and confidentiality in all interactions and demonstrating a commitment to maintaining the highest standards of professionalism.

Cultural competence: Awareness and respect for diverse cultures, fostering inclusivity in coaching relationships and the ability to navigate cultural differences and tailor coaching approaches accordingly.

Listening actively: Proficiency in listening actively, empathising with the client and creating a safe space that encourages clients to express themselves fully and in their preferred style.

Effective communication: Clear and concise communication to facilitate shared meaning, and support a sense of partnership between the mentor coach and the coach, prioritising the coach's development in relation to the core competencies.

EMCC

Reflective practice: Regular self-reflection to enhance personal and professional development. Encouraging coaches to engage in reflective practices for their own growth.

Holistic approach: Recognition of the interconnectedness of personal and professional aspects in a coach's life. Implementing a holistic coaching approach that addresses various dimensions of well-being.

Continual learning: Commitment to ongoing professional development, staying abreast of the latest coaching methodologies and practices. Encouraging coaches to embrace a mindset of continuous learning and improvement.

ICF and EMCC Mentor Coaching Duties and Responsibilities

ICF duties and responsibilities include:

Maintaining standards: Upholding the ICF Code of Ethics and Core Competencies by adhering to professional coaching standards to ensure quality and consistency.

Confidentiality: Safeguarding privacy and confidentiality to ensure a secure environment for open and honest communication.

Establishing the mentor coaching agreement: Collaboratively defining the coaching relationship, roles and expectations so as to ensure a mutual understanding of objectives and desired outcomes.

Co-creating the mentor coaching relationship: Establishing a partnership built on trust, open communication and a positive rapport, thus fostering an environment that promotes the mentor coaching client's self-discovery and growth.

Facilitating learning and growth as a professional coach: Employing effective mentor coaching techniques to support learning and growing of the ability to demonstrate core competency aligned coaching. Encouraging accountability and responsibility for the quality of coaching offered.

EMCC duties and responsibilities include:

Professional boundaries: Establishing clear boundaries to maintain a professional mentor coaching relationship. Recognising and addressing any potential conflicts of interest.

Evaluation and feedback: Providing constructive feedback to mentees on their developmental progress. Engaging in regular evaluations to assess the effectiveness of the mentor coaching offered.

Supportive challenge: Balancing support with challenging the mentee to explore new perspectives and possibilities. Nurturing a growth mindset through constructive feedback and encouragement.

Resource management: Identifying and leveraging resources for overcoming challenges. Facilitating access to networks and opportunities for professional development.

In summary, ICF and EMCC mentor coaches embody a unique set of characteristics, fulfil specific duties and have distinct responsibilities.

Blindspots and Bias in the Mentor Coaching

The ICF mentor coaching process is designed to be a robust and transformative experience. However, like any human interaction, the mentor coaching relationship is susceptible to blindspots and bias that can undermine its effectiveness. What are the blindspots and bias awareness issues that ICF mentor coaches need to be alive to noticing and managing?

Subjective Biases

Confirmation bias: The mentor coach may unintentionally seek or interpret information that confirms their pre-existing beliefs or assumptions about the mentor coaching client. This can limit the exploration of alternative perspectives and hinder the mentor coaching client's potential for growth that values their uniqueness, diversity and creativity.

Similarity bias: If the mentor coach and mentor coaching client share similar backgrounds or experiences, there is a risk of favouring those who are more similar, over those with more diverse perspectives and coaching styles. This bias may lead to a lack of inclusivity and hinder the mentor coach's ability to address the unique needs of individuals from different backgrounds. It can also impede the mentor coach from supporting the coach to develop ICF core competency aligned coaching that is fitting for the contexts in which they coach.

Halo effect: Positive traits or behaviours observed in one aspect of the mentor coaching client's coaching capability might overshadow noting the need for development in other areas. This bias can lead to overestimating overall capabilities, potentially depriving the mentor coaching client of getting what they need to support their development as a professional coach.

Objective Biases

Recency bias: Placing undue emphasis on the most recent interactions or achievements, whether positive or negative, may skew the feedback provided for a particular recording. This bias can cloud the mentor coach's ability to recognise sustained patterns of growth or challenges over time.

Availability bias: Giving more weight to readily available information about accomplishments or setbacks, without considering the broader context. This may lead to a narrow assessment of the mentor coaching client's capabilities and hinder the mentor coach's ability to provide even handed, expansive feedback.

Stereotyping: Making assumptions about a mentor coaching client based on stereotypes related to factors such as age, gender, language or cultural background. This arises in mentor coaching where mentor coaching clients with considerable life and coaching experience are expected to be more mature in their coaching, even when they have only recently started their credentialing learning journey. Coaches who are coaching in a language which is not their dominant language may be thought to be less capable at conducting a coaching conversation within recognisable and allowable variations of the ICF quality framework. This bias can contribute to a skewed response to a recording and limit the mentor coach's appreciation of the mentor coaching client's unique strengths.

Mitigating Biases in Mentor Coaching

There are a number of preventive and remedial actions that mentor coaches can take to manage the dilemmas that blindspots and bias can and do give rise to. These include but are not limited to:

Awareness raising via training: mentor coaches can participate in training to recognise and mitigate biases. Awareness of potential biases is the first step in minimising their impact.

Implementing a structured feedback process that focuses on specific competencies and behaviours can help counteract biases by ensuring a more fair evaluation.

Gathering input from multiple sources, including self-assessment and peer reviews, can provide a more comprehensive and balanced view of how well the mentor coach combines openness, flexibility and rigour.

Mentor coaches should engage in regular self-reflection to identify and address any emerging biases as they engage in reviewing coaching recordings and generating and providing feedback.

Acknowledging and addressing both subjective and objective biases is essential for mentor coaches to uphold the integrity of the mentor coaching process. By fostering an environment of self-awareness, ongoing learning and structured peer evaluation, mentor coaches can enhance the effectiveness and enjoyment of their mentor coaching work, despite it being ethically and labour intense.

A Solution Focused Approach to ICF Mentor Coaching in Action

ICF mentor coaching involves reviewing a piece of coaching in relation to the criteria of the ICF core competencies quality framework. The aim is to generate feedback that can be used in a coaching conversation with the mentor coaching client whose coaching is being reviewed.

ICF mentor coaching can be done in small groups (up to 10 participants), but at least 3 hours must be done individually with each credential applicant (International Coaching Federation, n.d. a). There are a variety of ways that mentor coaches structure the process of reviewing recordings. We will provide some of the common ways. This is not an exhaustive list and does not include the emerging trend to make use of AI-assisted transcript analyses.

Real Time vs Recorded Coaching

Mentor coaching can be offered in real time, i.e., the mentor coach observes a coaching session in real time and then immediately offers feedback, or the mentor coach reviews a recording submitted prior to the meeting for mentor coaching. With a recording, it is common for the mentor coach to require or invite the mentor coaching client to review their own recording as a way of becoming more familiar with the ICF core competency quality framework. It also encourages engaging autonomously with identifying strengths and developmental areas, as well as managing blindspots and bias.

To maintain a coaching mindset of openness, flexibility and curiosity, Solution Focused (SF) mentor coaches act as resource detectives, first focused on noticing and identifying where the core competencies are already detectable in the coaching. Note is taken about the unique style of the mentor coaching client and the ways they are making use of themselves as a person in their coaching while opening the space for full expression by their coaching client.

Partnering is fundamental to ICF's definition of coaching – "partnering in a thought-provoking and creative process that inspires them to maximise their personal and professional potential" (International Coaching Federation, n.d. b). Where a coach is applying a model in a scripted manner, with little responsiveness to the client's contribution to the conversation it is unlikely to be a passing recording for any of the ICF credentials. SF coaching and mentor coaching are characterised by co-creating.

The ICF provides criteria known as the Minimum Skills Requirements (International Coaching Federation, n.d. c) which allow the mentor coach and the mentor coaching client to anchor their observations when reviewing. This mitigates blindspots and bias and also promotes transparency and a partnering approach to learning and growth.

The SF mentor coach foregrounds the coach's growth and positions the ICF core competencies as a safety net – a resource to draw on when the coach is stuck, when there is insufficient progress between sessions or when there is a perception of insufficient value from the coaching. Rather than moving into deficit thinking, the SF mentor coach will listen for missed opportunities – moments where something different could be offered in the coaching session. The focus is held on the mentor coaching client's contributions. They are not blamed for what is happening/not happening in the coaching conversation, but rather are encouraged to be flexible and expansive about how to optimise their contributions.

Generating and Offering Feedback

Generating and offering feedback is an essential part of both ICF and EMCC mentor coaching. Offering effective mentor coaching feedback is seen as crucial for learning and growth. The SF mentor coach cultivates a context in which learning and growth rather than judgement and fault-finding provide sufficient safety to encourage exploration and experimentation. This increases awareness and a willingness to self-regulate the quality of one's coaching. Where coaching is not yet aligned with the ICF quality framework, mentor coaching supports the mentor coaching client to identify different ways to be and do in their coaching with the specific coaching client. Questions may include:

- "Let's suppose your coaching began to be more aligned with the core competency standards required, what might you notice yourself doing differently?"
- "What might that make possible for your client?"
- "What might you be drawing on in yourself when coaching in that way?"

Rather than delivering feedback as a set of observations as one might at the end of a performance evaluation, SF mentor coaches engage in a coaching conversation.

Generating feedback involves moving back and forth between the ICF core competencies and the coaching recording and its transcript. Audio recordings are used to check to what extent a piece of coaching meets the quality standard for a particular credential level. The transcript is used by the ICF mentor coach to select word for word examples from the coaching that demonstrate one or more markers/behaviourally anchored rating scales (BARS). This process makes it possible for a mentor coach and a mentor coaching client to compare the quality of coaching across a variety of recordings and to identify strengths and developmental areas.

Here is a step-by-step outline of how to generate SF feedback that is ICF aligned:

Lay the foundation for partnering: Establish through enquiry and exploration, the coach's desired outcome and best hopes for, and from the mentor coaching. This may include meeting specific ICF credentialing requirements, improving coaching skills or addressing particular areas of development related to the ICF core competencies. This is often done prior to a mentor coaching session and then checked to confirm or adjust during the mentor coaching session.

Adopt an open, curious mindset characterised by noticing in what ways the piece of coaching already meets the required standard. Be ready to catch any bias or blindspots, for example, are you bothered if a coach is coaching in a public space such as a coffee shop? Are you reactive when you hear the coach making use of a tool or technique that is not one that you hold in high regard or favour? Even simple self-checking questions help – for example, "at what time of day and under what circumstances am I at my most likely to do an even handed, fair job at reviewing a recording?"

Review the coaching session: Actively review the coaching session. Focus on the interplay between mentor coaching client and their coaching client. Look for the co-creation, the partnering. A way to do this is to consider 3–7 utterances at a time, rather than to review as if coaching is a question and answer language game.

Identify what the mentor coaching client is already doing well: Listening for presence or not absence of capability. Acknowledge and celebrate strengths, the effective use of coaching skills and alignment with the ICF core competencies. Feedback about where the coach shines reinforces good practices and builds confidence.

Identify developmental areas: Pinpoint specific areas where the mentor coaching client can improve or refine their coaching skills. This may involve identifying missed opportunities and noting any moments where the coaching is out of alignment with the ICF core competencies. Check that it is not bias but rather detectable misalignments which can be illustrated with extracts from the transcript.

Link feedback to the ICF core competencies: Provide criterion-referenced feedback, not opinion and preference. How do the observed coach contributions relate to specific competencies? Link feedback to examples. The transcript assists the mentor coach to do this efficiently, rather than needing to listen to the recording multiple times, or rely on memory if it was a real-time coaching session. By linking, the mentor coach supports the mentor coaching client to understand the connection between their coaching contributions and the ICF requirements.

Provide constructive feedback: Deliver feedback in a constructive and supportive manner. Use language that encourages growth and improvement rather than focusing solely on areas that need development. Offer specific examples to illustrate points and avoid generalisations. Stay close to the language choices of the mentor coaching client, rather than imposing your own preferences of expression.

Encourage self-reflection: Ask open-ended questions that prompt the mentor coaching coach to review their own coaching to identify areas for improvement and set developmental activities and signs of progress.

Agree on actionable next steps: Work collaboratively to design actionable next steps with detectable signs of progress. These should be aligned with the ICF core competencies and contribute to the coach's overall professional development.

Establish a plan for continued support: Co-develop a continuity promoting plan. Discuss how the mentor coaching client can experiment with the feedback in their coaching. Agree on the cadence of mentor coaching sessions to both allow for sufficient experimentation and integration, while maintaining momentum and optimism.

Document feedback: Document the feedback in such a way that it can serve as a reference for both throughout the mentor coaching relationship. Co-writing the notes and regarding the notes as owned by the mentor coaching client rather than the mentor coach is common in SF mentor coaching.

Review and Feedback: An Example

Here is an example of a mentor coach's reviewing of a coaching session. It starts with the synthesised feedback that the mentor coach prepared prior to meeting with the mentor coaching client. Then follows the annotated transcript used to generate the synthesised feedback. The numbers refer to the specific PCC markers that are detectable in this piece of coaching. You will see that one utterance by the coach may be demonstrating more than one core competency marker. We invite you to consider the following:

- What strengths do you detect in the mentor coaching client's style?
- If you were to be providing developmental feedback for this coach, what would be the 1–3 areas you would draw their attention to?

Extracts From the Annotated Transcript

Where you see ... this indicates that there is content that was not selected as an illustrative extract.

Coach:	00:22	Okay. So what are your best hopes from our session today? (3.1)
Client:	00:28	I think I need a little bit more clarity about my new role in the teams, I think. I think it would be good for me to get a little bit more details on how I could deal with that. (5.4)
Coach:	00:51	So clarity. How would you know that you have clarity? (3.2) (3.3) (5.1) (6.2)
Coach:	01:49	Okay, so get in touch with how you can do that. Okay. So what are you looking ... So what would you like to take away at the end of our session regarding this? (3.2) (3.3) (5.1) (5.4) (7.2) (7.7)
Client:	01:58	Take away. Maybe a little bit doubts and fears how others which ... how they see me or how they can interact with this role. (6.2) (6.3)

(Continued)

Coach:	02:16	Oh, okay. Take away, I thought … What are you going to take with you? (3.2) (3.3) (5.1) (5.4) (7.2)
Coach:	02:43	Okay. What would this good work result in, in the best case? (3.1) (5.4)
Client:	03:09	I think that we will have a lot of … not a lot of. But, certain meetings where we would talk about the next things to do, and what are our projects at the moment. I would know how to deal with all of this stuff. If they would like me to prioritise things, or if they would like to do it by their own, maybe. That would be good to know.
Coach:	03:49	Suppose you have that. What difference would that make to your life or their lives? Or your work? (3.3) (5.1) (6.5) (7.6)
Coach:	10:25	Okay. So correct me if I'm wrong, what you're looking for in this conversation is you want clarity around how you can work together as a team so … and how you can be a Product Owner so that in half a year or whichever time you work, still like working together. You have clarity around how decisions are made, how problems are talked about, et cetera, et cetera. (3.1) (3.2) (4.1) (6.7)
Client:	11:06	Yeah, that's right. Or the way how to get this clarity. Maybe that's enough.
Coach:	11:12	So if by the end of this session, you'd have some ideas around how to get this clarity – (3.2)
Client:	11:18	Yeah, right. That would be fine.
Coach:	11:27	Okay. Okay. Can I invite you to a little experiment. If this doesn't work for you, just push back, okay? (4.4) (5.3) (7.5)
Client:	11:35	Yeah, of course.
Coach:	27:20	So what gives you confidence that you can get there? (5.1) (8.5) (8.7)
Client:	27:26	I've already worked as a Product Owner, so I know this kind of role and what it is about. I know all the people in the team and I love them. That's great. So yeah, that's my four.
Coach:	30:46	How would this decision have to be so that it will give you confidence that, yes, we are on the right track? (5.2) (8.1) (8.3)
Coach:	32:30	What would you like to do? Would you like to kind of stay with this first step? Or would you go plan more steps after that one? (4.4) (5.3) (8.1) (8.6) (8.9)
Client:	32:42	No, to be honest, I think this first step would be a huge progress, because as I said, I think the structure thing is really important for our first stunt. For me, it would be great to have this first structure discussion with the team. Then, plan the next steps.
Coach:	33:10	Okay. So is there anything that you still want to discuss? With regard to your goal of being more clear what your role is and how this team is going to collaborate? Or are you good? (4.4) (8.9)
Client:	33:28	No, I think, yeah, for the moment I'm really good with it. It helped me a lot to talk about that now, I think it's not that a big problem. (5.3)
Coach:	33:43	Okay.
Client:	33:44	Yeah, it will be good. Thank you.
Coach:	33:47	Great, thank you so much. Brilliant. (4.2)

Synthesised Feedback

Main Strengths

CC3: Coaching Agreement

The coach demonstrated an understanding of exploring with the client towards the goal of the session. The coach asked questions to support the client to clarify what they wanted to see happening as a result of coaching, define measures of success and what needed to happen in the session. For example, the coach asked at minute 02:37 a clarifying question around the client's goal. The coach supported the client to clarify measures of success/ signs of progress for example, at minute 00:51.

CC4: Cultivates Trust & Safety

The coach most often asked clear questions, supporting the client to explore beyond the current perceptions and understanding of the situation. Plenty of examples at 08:10, 11:36, 3:21, 14:12, 14:51, 16:20, 17:40, 18:37, 22:05; "What difference would that make for you?", 15:20, 15:45, 22:54, 25:13.

Main Development Areas

CC5: Maintains Presence

The coach most often asked questions towards the exploration of "the what" – the situation that the client was describing. The coach could consider inviting the client into exploration of "the who" of the client. Examples of where the coach could have asked a question in that direction are at minutes 00:51, 02:16, 02:43, 01:49, 03:46, 13:21. This is a skill that the coach already exhibited at least once in the session at minute 22:05 "What difference would that make for you?".

CC7: Creating awareness and CC8: Facilitates client growth

The coach might consider exploring client learnings more so as to explicitly facilitate growth. Examples of questions that could be used include: "What are you becoming aware of about yourself today?" and "So, what did you learn in this session?"

Conclusion

Mentor coaching involves a variety of tasks and is a complex activity. It involves managing the paradox of having both more expertise in what professional coaching sounds like in relation to the ICF and EMCC quality frameworks, while simultaneously adopting a coaching mindset of appreciation, openness, flexibility and curiosity. It involves both rigour and creativity.

Useful Links

https://coachingfederation.org/credentials-and-standards/mentor-coaching
https://www.emccglobal.org/leadership-development/leadership-development-mentoring/
https://emccuk.org/Common/Uploaded%20files/Resources/supervision-techniques-03.pdf
https://www.emccglobal.org/leadership-development/supervision/competences/
ICF definition of coaching: https://coachingfederation.org/about
https://coachingfederation.org/credentials-and-standards/performance-evaluations/minimum-skills-requirements

References

EMCC Global. (n.d.). *Mentoring*. Retrieved February 7, 2024, from https://www.emccglobal.org/leadership-development/leadership-development-mentoring/
EMCC Global. (2019). *Supervision competence framework*. Retrieved from https://www.emccglobal.org/leadership-development/supervision/competences/
International Coaching Federation. (n.d. a). *Mentor coaching*. Retrieved February 7, 2024, from https://coachingfederation.org/credentials-and-standards/mentor-coaching
International Coaching Federation. (n.d. b). *What is coaching?* Retrieved February 7, 2024, from https://coachingfederation.org/about
International Coaching Federation. (n.d. c). *Minimum skills requirements*. Retrieved February 7, 2024, from https://coachingfederation.org/credentials-and-standards/performance-evaluations/minimum-skills-requirements
Lucas, M. (Ed) (2020). *Supervision techniques 3*. EMCC. Retrieved from https://emccuk.org/Common/Uploaded%20files/Resources/supervision-techniques-03.pdf

11 Coaching Supervision Groups

Jane Tuomola and Debbie Hogan

Introduction

Coaching supervision groups are often seen as a cost-effective way to provide coaching supervision, but this is only one of the many benefits of group coaching supervision as compared to individual coaching supervision. This chapter outlines the benefits as well as the challenges of coaching supervision groups and offers ideas for how to manage the challenges. The contracting process for how to set up a group is described, covering the aspects that are similar to setting up any individual coaching supervision contract as well as specific issues that need to be attended to in a group. Examples of Solution Focused (SF) questions are given to help the coaching supervisor enable the group to explore their best hopes for and from the group, as well as enabling the group to co-create roles within the group and take responsibility for their learning. The Solution Focused coaching supervision moves outlined earlier in the book are adapted to the context of coaching supervision groups. The Solution Focused reflecting team format for presenting cases in a group is outlined and includes a transcript of a group coaching supervision session using this process to bring this to life. Many coaching supervisors may feel nervous about supervising groups, so the chapter contains reflective exercises to help build the skills needed as a group coaching supervisor.

Hawkins and Schwenk (2006) list a number of guidelines for best practice in coaching supervision. One of these is that there should be a balance of individual, group and peer supervision as each has their limitations and so a mix of all optimises the benefits. As a supervisor, being aware of the benefits and challenges helps plan how to maximise the benefits and minimise the challenges.

Benefits and Challenges of Group Supervision

There are many benefits as well as challenges of group supervision, as compared to individual coaching supervision which apply no matter which model of supervision is being used (Butwell, 2006; Clutterbuck et al., 2016; Harrison & Bizouard, 2022; Lawrence, 2019; Proctor, 2008). These are summarised in Table 11.1.

DOI: 10.4324/9781003390527-11

Table 11.1 Benefits and Challenges of Group Supervision

Benefits of Group Supervision	Challenges of Group Supervision
• Economies of time, cost and expertise • Richer learning – breadth of client exposure • Networking/connections – builds a sense of community with those from the same professional background • Mutual support with others facing similar challenges • Interpersonal competencies • Shared and sharing of organisational knowledge • Vicarious learning – learning through listening and participating in colleagues' cases • Learning supervision skills • Greater diversity and quantity of feedback and reflections from multiple perspectives • Normalising common experiences – realising you are not alone and colleagues have similar challenges • Less likelihood of blind spots being missed than when there is one supervisor and one coach • Here and now experience of group life and systems dynamics that can potentially be transferred to work with clients/work settings • Puts challenges into perspective • Group dynamics if handled well can accelerate learning • Opportunity to experience other's coaching styles • Learning about yourself through being part of the group – how you see yourself, your reactions to others and their reactions to you	• Less individual time – not addressing needs • Confidentiality concerns (clients and supervisees) • Group dynamics can affect learning • Takes time to build up trust • Coaches can be more reluctant to self-disclose in a group setting for fear of feeling shame • Existing work relationships can get in the way and affect boundaries with co-workers • Structure of supervision may not mirror the process of coaching • Topics may be of limited relevance or interest to some members • Group dynamics if handled badly can impede learning • Attendance issues may impact the group • Lack of clarity on rules of engagement • Interpersonal conflict issues • Bringing personal issues to the group • Individuals voicing complaints or raising concerns privately to the supervisor • Diversity and cultural differences

Overcoming Challenges of Group Supervision

Dealing with challenges in group supervision requires skill, proactive strategies and commitment on the part of all the participants to facilitate a supportive and collaborative environment. We offer some approaches to address common challenges in group supervision:

- Establish clear ground rules and expectations generated by all the participants

  - Establish clear understanding and agreements related confidentiality and how information is shared within the group session and outside the session.

- Surface potential challenges and concerns from the group and establish clear agreements for how to manage them, i.e., conflict, tension, disagreements, how information is shared, attendance, participation, etc.

- Establish and maintain trust and rapport

  - Engage in group processes that facilitate building trust.
  - Allow time for members to get to know each other.
  - Model transparency and vulnerability.

- Facilitate group cohesion and ownership

  - Establish best hopes for and from group supervision.
  - Facilitate a group identity.
  - Take time to offer positive affirms to the group.
  - Invite the group to offer positive affirms to each other.

- Model respect and acceptance of diversity and cultural differences

  - Offer opportunities for members to comment on the added value of diversity and cultural contributions within the group.
  - Provide necessary support for members with unique needs.

- Provide opportunities for reflection, learnings and insights

  - Insure all voices are heard without judgement.

- Use a variety of facilitation skills to respect the learning needs of the individual

  - Individual reflection; small group process; open group discussion.

- Seek feedback and reflection

  - How satisfied are you with the process we're following?
  - How well does this process meet your expectations?
  - How satisfied are you with your growth and development from this process?
  - What changes, if any, would you suggest, to make it even better?

Types of Group Supervision

Proctor (2008, p. 32) identified four different types of group supervision:

- Authoritative (supervisor supervises each participant in turn and group members are mostly observers – referred to as supervision *in* a group)
- Participative (the supervisor takes the prime responsibility for supervising each member and also teaches and directs the members in co -supervising each other – referred to as supervision *with* the group)
- Cooperative (members agree to be active co-supervisors and takes responsibility for what they want from the group and how they would like to be

supervised; the supervisor still holds overall responsibility but takes a less active role – referred to as supervision *by* the group)
- Peer group supervision (no permanent supervisor, all participate equally in the role and responsibility of supervisor and supervision client)

SF group supervision fits best within the cooperative framework for a group. Peer supervision in a group will be discussed separately in Chapter 12.

Solution Focused Group Supervision

There has been nothing to date that we are aware of written about Solution Focused coaching supervision in groups. There are some articles on group supervision in the therapy space, which are outlined briefly below and then discussed in more detail at various points in the chapter where the ideas are relevant to group coaching supervision.

The most comprehensive writing on Solution Focused Supervision in the therapy space is by Thomas (2013). Group supervision is however a notable absence from the book except for one short section on the applications of supervision section of the book by Hsu and Kuo (2013) on Solution Focused supervision with school counsellors in Taiwan (pp. 197–204) which outlines the use of the reflecting team that is described in more detail later in this chapter.

Wheeler (2012) writes about transferring SF therapy ideas to supervision in a number of different formats for healthcare practitioners. He describes several SF questions and techniques that are useful for groups and are outlined below.

Tuomola (2017) wrote about her experience of becoming a group supervisor using the Solution Focused approach with two groups of case managers working at a psychiatric hospital. She shares using the reflecting team approach to case presentations, using role plays ("real plays") and SF questions to structure conversations on different topics. These ideas are all applicable to group coaching supervision and are described later in the chapter.

Bannink (2015) in her *Handbook of Positive Supervision (2015)* offers numerous exercises for SF supervisors that work in a group setting (described later). The book is aimed at any SF supervisor regardless of context so would also work well in group coaching supervision.

Starting any new supervision process begins with good contracting which is especially important in a group where there are many needs to be balanced.

Contracting in Group Supervision

Chapter 5 (see pp. 59–75) outlines the contracting process in individual supervision including the benefits of contracting, the practicalities and how to set up the psychological contract to create a safe space.

Before starting the contacting process, it is important to consider who is being brought together to attend the group, what brings them together, what are their preexisting relationships if any, what is the purpose of the group, how many people will attend and whether the group is open or closed. Often a supervisor may be contracted to supervise a group that already exists, such as a group of internal coaches or a group of coaches in the middle of coach training. If a supervisor wants to set up a group from scratch, the why, what, when and how of setting up a group are covered in Chapter 12 (see pp. 177–192) on peer supervision.

Many of the practicalities needing to be discussed in the contracting phase are identical for group supervision as they are for individual supervision such as venue, times of meeting, frequency, length of meeting, cancellation policy, confidentiality, payment and availability of the supervisor outside set times.

Clarifying the attendance expectations is important in a group. While individual supervision can be easily rearranged, the same is not true for a group so attendance expectations must be clarified at the start. The length of meetings is normally longer than individual supervision, although the frequency may be similar (often monthly).

The contracting may be two way, i.e. between the supervisor and group participants, or three way including an organisation, e.g. sponsoring a group of internal coaches to have supervision. There may be requirements from the organisation to take into account regarding the practicalities or confidentiality of the group. For example, does the organisation expect feedback on members participation or progress in the group? If so, this needs to be made clear at the start what the supervisor is expected to share and when.

We offer some Solution Focused questions as guidelines for contracting with a group.

Best Hopes From the Group

One of the challenges of group supervision is meeting both the needs of the individual as well as the needs of the group. Individual needs from the group can be discussed in the group using the best hopes question to build up a detailed picture of their preferred future:

- What are your individual best hopes **from** the group?
- What would you be noticing in your development as a coach as a result of us meeting?
- Who else would notice (clients, colleagues, your boss)?
- What would they be noticing?

While each person can be given equal time in the group, e.g. taking turns to present cases, these best hopes can be grouped into themes that are relevant to the majority of group members and can be prioritised when planning an overall agenda.

Including Other Stakeholders

As with all other SF conversation, bringing in outside perspectives can be helpful to explore how others would notice the supervision group has been helpful to the coach.

- How would your manager notice this supervision has been helpful to you?
- Who else in your organisation would notice?
- How would your clients notice you've been to this group?
- How would this group notice that you are making progress in your development as a coach?
- What would they be noticing?

Creative Ideas for Starting Supervision

A creative way of helping supervisees build on the discussion of best hopes in the group is to ask each member to write a supervision email from the future to the supervisor. This helps both clarify what changes they want to see in their coaching practice and what role they hope supervision to play in that development.

"It would be great if you could send me an email from a point in the future, in 6 months time, when you are looking back at the positive changes in your coaching practice in which you highlight how supervision has been useful in your practice".

Best Hopes for the Group/Ground Rules

The psychological contract is even more important in a group setting to set up a safe reflective space with clear rules on confidentiality and boundaries. As outlined in Chapter 5 (see pp. 59–75), this would include a discussion of the background of the supervisor (experience, expertise, working style), the background of the supervisees (their experience and learning needs), expectations of both the supervisor and supervisee, methods and models of supervision, specific workplace, ethical or legal issues to be aware of including dual roles, how feedback is given and how the group is reviewed.

When working in a group there needs to be a balance of group members' needs where "every voice needs to be heard as much as they want to be and serves the group".

Setting up ground rules for the group is an important part of this process. Unlike some other approaches where the group supervisor may specify the ground rules, in a Solution Focused group these are all co-constructed with the participants. As Wheeler and Richards (2007) outlines, this would typically take up the entire first meeting of the group – co-creating how the supervisor and group would work together. He shares that this often creates hopefulness about what the group has been designed to offer.

Some of the following questions can be a useful part of this process:

- What are your best hopes **for** the group so it has the highest potential of helping you towards your personal best hopes?
- What needs to happen in the group so that your best hopes come about?
- What are you hoping our group will be like?
- How would that show up in the ways we are with each other?
- What do you hope to be learning in this group?
- What will you be contributing to add value to this group?
- How can we **be** together so that everyone benefits and our time together is constructive and developmental?
- What else do we need to be aware of?
- How do we deal with challenges within the group?

Setting Up Group Supervision – Role of Supervisor

Wheeler and Richards (2007) suggests some questions that can be helpful to explore what the group expect the role of the supervisor to be:

- As you think about a typical meeting of this group, what do you imagine I will be doing?
- Suppose there was a video of the group, how would an observer be able to tell that I was the supervisor?
- From previous experiences of group supervision, what would you like me to do? What would you hope I don't do?

Setting Up Group Supervision – Sharing Responsibility for Learning

Clarifying expectations about who is responsible for learning is also important:

- How confident are you about taking responsibility for your own learning in this group?
- How will you let me know if we need to adjust the group process in any way?

Wheeler and Richards (2007, p. 359) shares a scaling question and how he used it with a group: "On a scale of 0 to 10 where 10 means I'm fully responsible for your practice development, and 0 means I have no responsibility at all, where's the number?" When the group produced a consensus around 5 he then asked "So, what do you need to be doing to make it as high as 5, and what do you want me to do so that its 5 and no higher?" This clarified that group members wanted scope to question each other and draw on each other's experience. They also wanted to draw on my practice experience which, for some, was more extensive than theirs. In response to the last point I negotiated that when I was asked what I would do in a particular practice situation

I might respond, "Yes, I have an idea about what I would do, but first can we see what other people might do?"

While the supervisor may bring many of these questions to the process of setting up the group, asking the group "What other questions come to mind that would be helpful in setting up the group successfully?" is also important.

Competence Frameworks in Relation to Group Supervision

The EMCC Supervision Competency Framework was outlined in Chapter 2, see pp. 7–27 (EMCC, 2019). Competence 8: Facilitates Supervision Groups relates specifically to group supervision and highlights the necessary skills in managing the dynamics of group supervision. It includes contracting to create a safe space, working in service of the group as a whole as well as the individuals within it, supporting the supervision group through stages of its development, adapting the process according to group dynamics, eliciting individual contributions, noticing and drawing attention to parallel process with this group and effectively managing time.

As discussed in Chapter 2 (see pp. 7–27), some of these ideas do not fit with the Solution Focused stance and need to be translated. For example, managing group dynamics positions the supervisor outside the group in an observational position. In SF that would be translated as "the ability to co-construct useful conversations within the group". As Dierolf and van der Hoorn state "In our view it is not necessary to surface and manage group dynamics to do that. In a situation in which a group is not serving the purpose of helping the individual supervision group members to grow, the Solution Focused supervisor would simply ask whether the group members are experiencing it similarly and what they would like instead" (Chapter 2, pp. 7–27).

As SF is a collaborative and co-constructed process, the supervisor invites the participants to observe and reflect on the dynamics, and what, if anything needs to be addressed in order for their growth and development to occur. The observations, impact and subsequent action is a shared reality versus the supervisor telling, giving or interpreting the situation from an "expert stance". Managing the group process from a Solution Focused Perspective is explored more below.

Group Process From a Solution Focused Perspective

A Solution Focused group process differs from traditional group process in the philosophical orientation, the management of goal setting and how change is facilitated within a group.

Philosophical Orientation

- Traditional group process is based on psychological theories and focuses on exploring the unconscious dynamics to develop insight and self-awareness. It requires the facilitator to have training and knowledge about group dynamics and its impact on the individual and group psyche.

- Solution Focused group process is rooted in the principles discussed in Chapter 3 (see pp. 27–42) which is oriented to the resources, capability and expertise of all the individuals involved. They are part of the co-construction and meaning making of the interactions within the group and its impact on the individual and the group.

Goal Orientation

- Traditional group process focuses on the underlying psychological issues and interpersonal dynamics within the group and uses psychological theory as a lens in which to interpret these dynamics.
- Solution Focused group process is goal-oriented and future focused. It engages in the desired outcome and hopeful change, and co-constructs small actionable steps in the direction of what is wanted rather than dwelling on the past problems and events.

Facilitating Change

- Traditional group process focuses on gaining insight and emotional processing by exploring the problematic past and the impact of the events on the present.
- Solution Focused group process focuses on identifying and utilising the person's past and present capabilities and as resources for achieving the success they desire for the present and hopeful future.

Sharry, J. (2007). Solution-Focused Groupwork. London: Sage offers some useful ideas about how to manage group process from a Solution Focused Perspective based on therapy groups. These ideas would also be applicable to group supervision. He advises aiming for the right balance between three things:

Solution Talk Versus Problem Talk

Sharry states that the content of the group affects the process. By keeping the emphasis on goals, exceptions, strengths and what is going right, the content is light, energetic and focused on creativity. What facilitators draw attention to and what they ensure gets group time powerfully influences the content and quality of the group process – the supervisor needs to be aware that this includes nonverbal reinforcement of solution talk. However problem talk is not always undesirable –it can be a relief to know that you are not the only coach struggling with something and can provide some motivation for change. Sometimes it can helpful to invite problem talk, e.g. if many of group are expressing positive successes, others who are struggling may feel silenced and stop contributing unless invited. Too much problem talk can however become unhelpful, e.g. increasing sharing of despair or blame and hostility towards other group members. The aim is about balance – Sharry suggests aiming for about 80% solution talk and 20% problem talk.

Group-Centred Interactions Versus Facilitator Centred Interactions

The supervisor needs to encourage group members to interact with each other not just with the facilitator although this can take time to build up. Initially in new groups there can be a higher dependence on the group members looking to the facilitator for guidance. Enabling group-centred interactions allows members to derive powerful support and have access and idea and solutions from each other. It helps them take more responsibility to ensure the group fits with their needs and wishes. There are times when the facilitator needs to take control of the process such as establishing confidentiality and group rules, ensuring the group starts and finishes on time, ensuring the agenda is covered, helping quiet people contribute, not allowing one person to dominate and moderating group conversation to ensure it is balanced. At other times the supervisor must sit back and allow the group to take the lead.

Client-Generated Solutions Versus Supervision-Generated Solutions

The role of the facilitator is to ensure the balance between ideas the group generates themselves and supervisor-generated solutions. The effectiveness of the group will be severely limited if group members simply take what the supervisor may suggest without challenging the ideas and adapting them to their specific context.

Solution Focused Supervision Moves in Group Supervision

Once the group is formed, and there is a good contract in place, the following tools can be useful in the ongoing supervision sessions: Solution Focused moves from the art gallery metaphor, the reflecting team approach to presenting cases as well as other ways of making use of the group such as role plays. Each of these are discussed below.

Applying Solution Focused Supervision Moves to Group Supervision

The SF supervision moves from the art gallery metaphor were discussed in Chapter 4 (see Figure 4.1). The same moves can also be applied in group supervision. Each session should start with the "ticket office", i.e. planning the agenda for the session. This helps keep the focus and effectively manages the time for the session (EMCC, 2019).

Each SF group supervision session starts off with everyone sharing what has been going well since the last meeting (similar to asking coaching clients what has been better since the last meeting).

There is evidence from organisational psychology of the positive impact this Solution Focused way of starting a group can have. "People think better throughout the whole meeting if the very first thing they do is to say something true and positive about how their work or the work of the group is going" (Kline, 1999, p. 107). Additional research found that not only was "resource activation" required for good outcomes in therapy, but that "successful therapists ... focused on their clients' strengths from the very start of a therapy session" (Gassman & Grawe, 2006). Hence it is likely that this would also be true in supervision.

After that, the group plans the agenda for the session which could include:

- 1–2 case presentations
- Topic discussions
- Role plays
- Sharing ideas from reading/resources

Once the overall agenda for the session has been planned, for each topic on the supervision agenda, the SF supervision moves gallery can be used to guide the discussion. Each coach can share their ideas in turn, and the picture that is created by the group is often richer than it would be then by any one coach alone. These are some examples of questions that can be used.

Ticket Office

- What would you like to come out of our supervision discussion on this topic today so that it is helpful for you?

Preferred Future Gallery

- Suppose you have all the knowledge and skills you need in this area, what would you be noticing? How would you be showing up when you are the coach you want to be in this area?
- What would your clients/colleagues be noticing? How would they respond?
- What difference would this make to you?

Successful and Past Instances Gallery

- What do you already know about this topic?
- What are you already doing well in this area? What do your clients/colleagues notice?
- On a scale of 1–10, how confident are you in this area?
- What has got you to that number and not lower? What else ....

For each question, the aim is to get a rich detailed description of the skills, knowledge and resources the coach already has, which they can then use to help them move even further forwards.

As the supervision is coming to a close the following questions from the Gift Shop part of the SF moves gallery can help the coaches think about learning from the session and next steps

Gift Shop

- How will you know when you are one point higher on this scale? What would be some small concrete signs of progress in this area?
- What will your clients/colleagues notice you doing differently?
- What did you learn from the discussion – about the topic/about yourself as a coach?
- What was helpful from the reading/discussion?
- What questions do you still have (then either answered by the group, or discussed how they would go about finding the answers)?
- What would you like to experiment with in relation to this before our next supervision session?
- How will you take these ideas forwards in your own practice?
- What are your next small steps to take in this area so you can move up your scale?

Reflecting Team Model of Case Presentations in a Group

In addition to the Solution Focused moves above, using reflecting teams can be helpful in group supervision. The idea of a reflecting team was originally written about by Andersen (1987, 1991). Norman (2003) later adapted the ideas and wrote about Solution Focused reflecting teams. He described this way of using the reflection team in relation to supervision of therapists. The wording here has therefore been changed slightly to be applicable to coaches.

The reflecting team is most often used as a way of a coach presenting a case in the group where they are struggling and would like help to move forwards. The presenting coach can also bring other areas of their practice that they would like to develop.

Preparing

The coach who wishes to reflect on a piece of their coaching practice comes to the meeting with a request for exploration around a specific practice issue. Before sharing anything about the client, they state what their best hopes from the discussion are.

Presenting

The coach outlines their request and offers relevant information to the team about the situation. Members of the team listen attentively and let the coach finish without interruption.

Clarifying

The team asks questions to clarify so as to have sufficient understanding of the coach's best hopes and the situation so as to be able to respond to the coach's request to the team. These questions are for clarification only – questions implying guidance such as "Have you tried ..." are not allowed.

Affirming

The team members each offer the coach what most impressed each of them about how the coach is handling themselves and the situation. The coach listens silently to each item of feedback and says "Thank you" graciously to each one.

Reflecting

Going round, the team members take it in turn to offer one observation or appropriate comment at a time. What is offered may be anything the team member thinks relevant and beneficial, e.g. technical input, advice, reflections, metaphors, poetry, jokes, etc. If someone has nothing to offer, they say "Pass" and the cycle continues until everyone has said all they want to say, or time has run out. The benefit of reflecting in this way is that the inputs tend to build creatively on each other.

During this phase, the coach remains silent and listens. He/she may take notes.

Closing

When all the reflections have been made, the coach responds briefly to what has been said, thanks everyone and summarises/synthesises what they are taking away as awareness and learning generated from the reflections. They include a statement about how they will apply this to improve/benefit their coaching practice.

The value of this process is that the coaches in the group do not have to use the Solution Focused approach in their own work to benefit. The aim of the process is to listen to and offer ideas based on what the presenting coach wants from the discussion. It fits with the tenets of the model being pragmatic (exploring and moving towards what is wanted) and respectful as the coach is not being told what to do, but offered ideas that they decide how they want to take forwards.

The listeners are listening in a Solution Focused way, i.e. listening to give positive feedback and listening for exceptions, goals and preferred futures. The group is not listening to analyse the coach or their client. The affirming comments invite the coach to expand their awareness of their abilities (Norman, 2003).

The supervisor would normally be the facilitator of this process, keeping track of time and making sure everyone in the group takes turns to answer. However, as the group evolves and the coaches become familiar with the process, the group members can also take turns as facilitators.

One coach explains the positive impact of the reflecting team approach in group supervision (J. Davies, personal communication, January 18, 2022):

> Invaluable learning using the reflecting team format, where I was actively participating as well as listening to the reflections of other colleagues. The experience was truly enriching to broaden my own way of thinking and questioning for my own clients. Developing the confidence to present a case to the group, who was able to support me to think from different perspectives about the same issue that I have been struggling with alone. I walked away feeling lighter, unstuck and more possibilities to work with my clients.

Appendix (see p. XXX) shows a transcript from a group supervision session using the reflecting team format. In this example the supervisor acts as a facilitator only. However, more often the supervisor would also share affirmations and reflections.

As you read the transcript answer some of the following questions:

- What are you noticing about the stance of the process?
- What did that make possible for the person?
- What skills do you already have that would enable you to do this process well?
- Where would you need to develop?
- What might have been helpful from the presenter's point of view?
- What might have been helpful for the participants' point of view?
- What did you learn? What surprised you?

Skills Practice – Making Use of the Group

Following any case presentation or topic discussion, the group can also try out the ideas immediately through the use of role plays (playing the client just discussed) or real plays (trying out an idea with the coachee bringing a real topic of their own to the conversation) as described in Tuomola (2017).

The value of groups is that there are so many options. The role plays can be done in pairs and learning is discussed as a group, or the role play is done in front of the group and the group feeds back what went well and suggests ideas for what could be even better.

Bannink (2015) describes many other creative exercises that can make use of the group format to find competence such as group members interviewing each other about satisfaction and capabilities (p. 74); positive gossip (p. 77) where group members can be invited to take turns to positively gossip about each other; and creating an appreciation wall (p. 79), where each group member writes on a sheet of paper what they appreciate about their colleagues. These exercises are a way of both increasing the supervision client's competence and a way of utilising the group to practice SF skills that they in turn can use with their clients.

Reviewing the Group

As outlined in Chapter 8 on deliberate practice, seeking regular feedback from clients increases therapists (and coaches) effectiveness and is one of the factors that can lead to becoming a "super shrink" (see pp. 111–124). Bannink (2015, p. 114) outlines the similar process with supervisors who ask for regular feedback helping supervisors adjust supervision to what is important to their supervision clients and become "super-supervisors".

Chapter 8 discussed the concept of deliberate practice using the Outcome Rating Scale (ORS, Miller & Duncan, 2000) to rate client's progress in coaching and how the sessions are using the Session Rating Scale (SRS, Miller et al., 2002). There is also a Group Session Rating Scale (GSRS, Duncan & Miller, 2007) that can be used at the end of each group supervision session to review how each individual is finding the group (see Figure 11.1).

The GSRS is available for use by individual clinicians at no cost as long as they register for a free licence here: http://scott-d-miller-ph-d.myshopify. com/collections/performance-metrics/products/performance-metrics-licenses-for-the-ors-and-srs.

Each group member is asked to rate the group on the four scales of relationship, goals and topics, approach or method and overall. Whatever the score, the supervisor can ask what they can do differently or better the next time to get an even higher score. When the scores are already high the supervisor can ask what they need to continue doing to maintain the high scores.

This can be used along with other SF questions to review the group in detail as outlined by Bannink (2015, p. 112).

- If 10 stands for the optimal functioning of our group and 0 stands for the opposite, where do I think the group stands today?
- How is it that the functioning of the group is at this point on the scale and not lower?
- What do we want to keep as it is and doesn't need to change?
- At what point on the scale would I like our group to be in future?
- How will one point higher look? What will we be doing differently or better?
- What will be signs of further progress?
- How can we get a higher point on the scale?
- Who will do what and when to make that happen?
- How are we going to celebrate progress?

The process of reviewing the group can also be created collaboratively with the group. For example, asking:

- How often do we want to review how our group is going?
- How would you like to review our group?
- What questions do we need to be asking to review our group?

The combination of good contracting at the beginning of a group and regularly reviewing what is working and what could be even better helps minimise

Group Session Rating Scale (GSRS)

Name _____ Age (Yrs):____
ID# _____ Gender_____
Session # ____ Date: _____

Please rate today's group by placing a mark on the line nearest to the description that best
fits your experience.

Relationship

I did not feel understood,   I felt understood,
respected, and/or   I--I   respected, and
accepted by the leader   accepted by the leader
and/or the group.   and the group.

Goals and Topics

We did *not* work on or   We worked on and
talk about what I   I--I   talked about what I
wanted to work on and   wanted to work on and
talk about.   talk about.

Approach or Method

The leader and/or the   The leader and
group's approach is a   I--I   group's approach is a
not a good fit for me.   good fit for me.

Overall

There was something   Overall, today's group
missing in group   I--I   was right for me—I felt
today—I did not feel   like a part of the group.
like a part of the group.

International Center for Clinical Excellence

www.centerforclinicalexcellence.com
www.scottdmiller.com

© 2007, Barry L. Duncan and Scott D. Miller

To obtain full working copies of these measures, please register online at:
http://www.scottdmiller.com/node/13

Figure 11.1 The Group Session Rating Scale (Duncan & Miller, 2007) (Reproduced
    with permission)

the challenges outlined at the start of the chapter and ensures they are addressed as soon as possible.

Reflective Exercise – Developing the Skills of a Group Supervisor

Moving from offering individual supervision to group supervision can be
daunting as outlined in Tuomola (2017). Below is a reflective exercise adapted

from Rebolj and Iveson (2021) in a course on Solution Focused Groupwork that can also be used for those wanting to become a group supervisor or improve their skills as a group supervisor. This can be done alone, by asking yourself the questions or done with a partner where you interview each other.

- List all the skills you think a group supervisor would need and then answer the following questions:
  - Pick a skill from the list where you would rate yourself above a 7 and ask: How did you get good at this skill? What did it take to develop this skill? How does this skill show up? How do others notice this?
  - Pick a skill where you are at a 4 or 5 and ask suppose you had even more of this skill what would be different? What would you notice? What would others notice?
  - Pick a skill where you are below a 2 and ask what gives you hope that this seed has already been planted?

References

Andersen, T. (1987). The reflecting team: Dialogue and meta-dialogue in clinical work. *Family Process, 26,* 415–428.

Andersen, T. (Ed.). (1991). *The Reflecting Team: Dialogues and Dialogues about the Dialogues.* W.W. Norton.

Bannink, F. (2015). *Handbook of Positive Supervision for Supervisors, Facilitators, and Peer Groups.* Hogrefe Publishing GmbH.

Butwell, J. (2006). Group supervision for coaches: Is it worthwhile? A study of the process in a major professional organisation. *International Journal of Evidence Based Coaching and Mentoring, 4*(2), 43–53.

Clutterbuck, D., Whitaker, C., & Lucas, M. (2016). *Coaching Supervision: A Practical Guide for Supervisees.* Routledge.

Duncan, B.L., & Miller, S.D. (2007). *The group session rating scale.* Author. Retrieved from http://scott-d-miller-ph-d.myshopify.com/collections/performance-metrics/products/performance-metrics-licenses-for-the-ors-and-srs

European Mentoring Coaching Council [EMCC] (2019, June). *Supervision competence framework.* European Mentoring Coaching Council. https://www.emc-cglobal.org/leadership-development/supervision/competences/

Gassman, D., & Grawe, K. (2006). General change mechanisms: The relation between problem activation and resource activation in successful and unsuccessful therapeutic interactions. *Clinical Psychology and Psychotherapy, 13*(1), 1–11.

Harrison, L., & Bizouard, M. (2022). The magic of group supervision. In F. Campone, J. DiGirolamo, D. Goldvarg & L. Seto (Eds.). *Coaching Supervision: Voices from the Americas* (pp. 168–183). Routledge.

Hawkins, P., & Schwenk, G. (2006). *Coaching Supervision: Maximising the Potential of Coaching.* Chartered Institute of Personnel and Development.

Hsu, W.S., & Kuo, B.C.H. (2013). Solution-focused supervision with school counselors in Taiwan. In F. Thomas (Ed.). *Solution-Focused Supervision. A Resource Oriented Approach to Developing Clinical Expertise* (pp. 197–204). Springer.

Kline, N. (1999). *Time to Think: Listening to Ignite the Human Mind.* Hachette.

Lawrence, P. (2019). What happens in group supervision? Exploring current practice in Australia. *International Journal of Evidence Based Coaching and Mentoring, 17*(2), 138–157.

Miller, S.D., & Duncan, B.L. (2000). *The Outcome Rating Scale*. Author.

Miller, S.D., Duncan, B.L., & Johnson, L.D. (2002). *The Session Rating Scale 3.0*. Author.

Norman, H. (2003). Solution focused reflecting teams. In W. O'Connell & S. Palmer (Eds.). *Handbook of Solution-Focused Therapy* (pp. 156–167). Sage Publications.

Proctor, B. (2008). *Group Supervision*. Sage Publications.

Rebolj, B., & Iveson, C. (2021, April 15–16). Solution focused group workshop. [Course presentation]. BRIEF.

Thomas, F.N. (2013). *Solution-Focused Supervision. A Resource Oriented Approach to Developing Clinical Expertise*. Springer.

Tuomola, J. (2017). From the blind leading the blind to leading from one step behind: Experiences with running a solution focused supervision group for case managers. In D. Hogan, D. Hogan, J. Tuomola & A.K.L. Yeo (Eds.). *Solution Focused Practice in Asia* (pp. 90–94). Routledge.

Wheeler, J. (2012). Solution focused supervision. In T.S. Nelson & F.N. Thomas (Eds.). *Handbook of Solution Focused Brief Therapy. Clinical Applications*. Routledge.

Wheeler, S., & Richards, K. (2007). The impact of clinical supervision on counsellors and therapists, their practice and their clients: A systematic review of the literature. *Counselling and Psychotherapy Research*, 7(1), 54–65.

12 Peer Coaching Supervision and Intervision

Jane Tuomola and Debbie Hogan

Introduction

The terms "peer coaching supervision" and "intervision" are both used to describe a peer-led group engaged by coaches who each contribute knowledge, skills and experience and support each other to learn and grow from one another's coaching practice. There is no designated leader, rather a sense of equity, commitment to generating benefit for all and self-organisation are characteristic of the fabric of these groups. This chapter starts by outlining the differences inherent in these names – "supervision" implying vision from above, compared with "intervision" meaning between, among, reciprocally or together. Peer supervision can occur in reciprocal pairs or a peer supervision chain process as well as in a group format. The benefits and challenges of this form of coaching supervision are discussed, using examples of Solution Focused (SF) questions to help maximise the benefits and minimise the challenges. The process of co-creating a well-functioning peer supervision process is outlined including establishing the "why" or purpose of the group, followed by the what, when, where and how. Examples of peer supervision groups in action are shared.

What's in a Name? Some Definitions

Peer supervision differs from the forms of supervisor led supervision discussed earlier in this book. It refers to the reciprocal arrangements where peers work together for mutual benefit and more self-directed learning is emphasised (McNicoll, 2008). Before exploring this in more detail it can be useful to look at some definitions.

A peer is defined as: "a person of the same age, the same social position, or having the same abilities as other people in a group" (Cambridge Dictionary, n.d.). In the context of peer coaching supervision, this means coaches who would have a similar level of skills, knowledge or ability – so there is a sense of equality or collegiality.

While the term peer supervision is commonly used, other coaches use the word intervision to refer to this process. Supervision literally means vision

DOI: 10.4324/9781003390527-12

from above whereas intervision means vision among or between. Some ideas are shared below regarding these two terms.

Turner and colleagues in their comprehensive book on Peer Supervision in Coaching and Mentoring found the following as a starting point for the definition of peer supervision: "two or more coaches seek to assist each other in reflecting on their practice including both case specific and coach specific reflection" (Standards Australia, 2011, as cited in Turner et al., 2018, p. 9).

They broadened this to define peer supervision as a "collaborative learning environment created between fellow coaches, mentors or other professionals (practitioners). It is of mutual benefit to the practitioners involved as well as being of service to their clients and the wider system" (Turner et al., 2018, p. 7).

Martin et al. (2017) offer a critique of the terminology "peer group supervision" in health care settings. They state that peer group supervision is intended to foster safe and effective practice, through providing informal, reciprocal collegial assistance with group members related to clinical and professional concerns. However, in peer group supervision no one has the authority over other group members and therefore "no member should monitor, evaluate, direct or assume clinical responsibility for the other group members". They therefore see this term as an oxymoron as one of the defining functions of supervision both logically and legally is monitoring and directing the work of the supervision client. They even state that it is somewhat fraudulent as it implies supervision is in place when it is not. Instead, they suggest peer group supervision is not suitable for trainees or novice practitioners and should be labelled peer consultation and supplemented by formal supervision with a supervisor.

In the coaching landscape, these same concerns have been shared about peer supervision being an oxymoron, as it implies one coach has the vision over the other. Therefore in some parts of the world this is referred to as intervision instead as this involves learning from others and seeing them and their work from within, together and mutually. Intervision has been defined as: "a supervision process involving a group of peers with the same professional focus, who co-operate in a goal-driven process towards finding solutions within a shared structural design. Mutually accountable volunteers give and receive learning and teaching without compensation" (Lippmann, 2009).

"Intervision is based on the idea that you alone are ultimately responsible for your own behaviour. You learn to look differently at yourself, at what you do and search for things to improve. In intervision you take charge of your professional development, your expertise in your field, the way you work with others and your personal performance" (Bellerson and Kohlman, 2016, p. 9).

Neither of these terms however is specific to the approach or model that is being used in the process. Bannink (2015, p. 15) shares that most definitions of peer supervision are either problem focused or neutral in their wording. She offers a definition of positive peer supervision as "building solutions among peers for greater personal and methodical competence with support and encouragement to and from each other in discussing and implementing these skills".

While there are concerns about the term peer supervision, as this is still the more widely used terminology, peer supervision will be used throughout this chapter when referring to supervision that is not supervisor led.

Who Can Take Part in Peer Supervision

Turner et al. (2018, p. 7) define that peer supervision is between two more people who have not been trained as supervisors. They argue that once coaches train as supervisors, then the work would move out of the domain of peer supervision into professional supervision even if no money changes hands.

Other authors do not make this distinction and write about their experiences in peer supervision groups between coaches who are all trained as coaching supervisors but meeting as peers in the supervision space (e.g. Pliopas, 2021; Udale & Routt, 2021).

As we see it, the important factor is that the pair or group is made up of people who consider themselves as peers according to the definition above where the coaches share a similar level of knowledge, skills and experience, and this may include training as a coaching supervisor.

Why Choose Peer Supervision?

There can be many reasons coaches choose to engage in peer supervision which may be instead of or in addition to supervisor led supervision.

Some of the reasons a group of coaches on a recent coaching supervision course (SolutionsAcademy, 2023) gave for participating in peer supervision groups rather than a supervisor-led supervision process included:

- "It's cheaper" and "makes the most value of existing resources in the system"
- "No fears of inadequacy; I like the democratic space"
- "Excited to work with peers I respect"
- "Informal setting, no power differentials"
- "Mutual support and empowerment – we rotate the role of facilitator so we all get to learn"
- "Shared leadership"

These mirror the benefits shared in the literature (e.g. Clutterbuck et al., 2016; McNicoll, 2008; Turner et al., 2018):

- Cost effective as time rather than money is exchanged
- Increased access and frequency of supervision which has an overall benefit to clients
- Increased skills and responsibility for self-assessment and decreased dependency on expert supervisors
- Sense of power can be diluted which deepens the sense of personal responsibility in the supervision client

Reduce the sense of isolation as an independent practitioner

- When in the supervisor role you can gain valuable feedback on your facilitation skills
- Useful sounding board to decide whether a particular issue needs to be taken to a qualified supervisor
- Those with lower confidence may feel more comfortable working with someone with a similar level of experience
- Easier to be vulnerable with someone also bringing their own struggles
- Connecting with peers locally is often logistically simpler due to the shortage of coaching supervisors
- A natural place to continue to develop skills among a group of alumni from a training course – existing camaraderie adds to the depth of rapport and connection as well as having a shared philosophy of practice
- Someone on the same level to benchmark your practice with

These benefits make peer supervision a valuable adjunct or alternative to regular supervision. The benefits can be increased if the group uses robust and well-designed supervision tools and there are enough members in the group to offer diverse perspectives and account for any potential deficits in knowledge (McNicoll, 2008).

Challenges of Peer Supervision

There can however be numerous challenges in peer supervision which include the following (Clutterbuck et al., 2016; McNicoll, 2008; Turner et al., 2018):

- Process may be seen as eliminating the need for other forms of professional supervision.
- The more collegial type of relationship can lead to cosiness or collusion (I won't challenge you if you don't challenge me).
- Discussions may focus more on techniques and business development than client safety and become peer coaching rather than peer supervision.
- Not all professional bodies recognise peer supervision for the purposes of accreditation.
- It works less well when the coaches are less experienced as there is insufficient breadth of experienced to generate problem solving.
- Disorientation and confusion (feeling undermined by others or confused by what you hear but not having the confidence to ask for clarification).
- Discounting your own experience (feeling in awe of others and not sharing your experience).
- Developmental stagnation – working with people you trained with who all see things in a similar way and lack multiple perspectives.
- Minimising your own supervision needs (giving more than you are getting but not speaking up).

- Comparisons with peers breeding competitiveness.
- Dual relationships/conflicts of interest if pre-existing relationships exist.
- Dependency or overinvesting (starting to outgrow the relationship but feeling trapped, especially if few other options for supervision locally or invested too much to walk away).
- Lack of ownership (not everyone fully engages in the process).

These benefits and challenges are relevant whether the peer supervision is done as one to one or as a group. However, there are additional benefits and challenges depending on the form of the peer supervision which are outlined below (Clutterbuck et al., 2016; Turner et al., 2018).

Forms of Peer Supervision

One to One Peer Supervision

Peer supervision can take the format of two coaches meeting and taking it in turns to supervise each other. The benefits of one to one or reciprocal peer supervision include being clear who is holding the space and who is the client (who is responsible for how to use the time), that there is dedicated time for personal reflection, it is possible to notice patterns and development over time and that this can be more easily arranged on an ad hoc basis. This arrangement works well when the two coaches are at a similar developmental stage as each may feel more open to sharing concerns about their work without feeling judged by someone with more experience.

The limitations may be that the one in the supervisor role may not be able to offer a breadth of perspectives, there could be a mutual dependency which may be unhealthy if not managed properly, unhelpful patterns may go unnoticed and the experience may be unbalanced if one peer lacks expertise.

Peer Supervision Chain

Instead of two coaches providing reciprocal supervision to each other, some coaches have set up what is known as a peer supervision chain. This is where a group of coaches enter into an arrangement where each agrees to supervise and be supervised on a rotational basis. For example, person A supervises person B, person B supervises person C and person C supervises person A. Every few months the rotation of who supervises whom changes. Each chain member is therefore both a supervisor and supervision client and gets to experience a range of supervision styles.

Udale and Routt (2021) write about their peer supervision chain which at times contained up to 20 members and, in addition to the individual supervision sessions, met as a group to review learnings. Benefits they found included the rich experience from working with a number of different supervisors over time and the safety each felt for having the opportunity to practice and explore different techniques in a safe setting. They found some challenges during the process and offer some learnings to others considering this way of working, such as the importance of good contracting within each dyad, agreeing on a feedback process, declaring a shared commitment to the process and a willingness to experiment. The administrative load also needed acknowledging and managing.

Using the ideas outlined in Chapter 4 on individual supervision, Chapter 5 on ethics and contracting and Chapter 6 on case supervision are all relevant for creating a well-functioning one-to-one peer supervision relationship. Discussing these challenges beforehand such as how to give feedback, where else to go for support if an issue can't be resolved through the peer conversation and how often and how to review the supervision so that it remains helpful to both parties can help minimise some of these challenges.

Peer Group Supervision

Peer supervision can also take place in a group. Many of the benefits of peer group supervision are similar to the benefits outlined in Chapter 11 for group supervision with a supervisor (see pp. 159–177). Additional ones for peer group supervision in a group include having a high level of understanding and support for each other's developmental needs and learning group supervision skills by taking turns in the facilitator role.

Proctor (2008, p. 127) shares a great quote that the "the peer group needs to be leaderful rather than leaderless" and is a place where all members need to develop both the skills of supervisor and supervision client. She sees peer group supervision as potentially groundbreaking, as it is a place to learn how to give authority to others as appropriate and learn how to take authority gracefully.

The specific challenges of peer supervision in a group are listed below (Clutterbuck et al., 2016; McNicoll, 2008; Turner et al., 2018):

- Groups can lack structure and degenerate into chat/gossip/discussion groups.
- Demands on people's time can impact attendance – easy to miss when not paying.
- Skills in the group may not be enough to handle the supervisory issues involved.
- The process could become diluted and collusion can be rife.
- Boundaries may be harder to maintain and easy to get off track without a supervisor.
- Individuals may dominate or become passive and group dynamics may impact on the group – and no one takes responsibility for addressing the issues.
- If the group is connected through the same course, there may be blind spots due to the homogeneity of the group.

- The group may have varying levels of capability in managing group dynamics.
- Set up could take longer without one person being in charge of the contracting.
- Group think. Members feel pressured to maintain unity of the group.
- Different levels of expertise – so members defer to those more experienced.

While there are numerous challenges, as one coach commented "it's possible to have a really well functioning peer group and supervisor led supervision being really unhelpful" (SolutionsAcademy, 2023).

Factors for Effective Peer Group Supervision

The rest of the chapter will focus on what factors are important in facilitating effective peer group supervision and how this can be done using an SF approach.

The following factors have been found to contribute to effective peer group supervision (McNicoll, 2008; Turner et al., 2018):

- Equality – members need to feel free to speak about their practice so the group should be made up of peers where no one has more or less status by way of seniority or experience.
- Supportive Culture – people need to feel safe and free from judgement and the assumptions that people do their best with the resources they have and to acknowledge that its ok to make mistakes.
- Structure – the supervision sessions need to be well structured to create safety and boundaries.
- Value on attendance – members need to commit to the group and make it a priority, scheduled in advance ideally for a year.
- A formal commitment with a written contract, which has been co-created collectively, reviewed regularly and re-contracted as required.
- Super + vision – ensure the supervision is high quality, that there is a balance of positive and challenging feedback and that the aim is to promote useful self-reflection for the supervision client.
- Self-directed – supervision clients need to be self-directed learners, determining their own supervision needs and the group need to focus on the benefit for the supervision client offering resources and insightful solutions.
- No post mortems – no further discussion of what happens in the group outside the group to contribute to the group feeling safe.
- Access to external professional supervision either individually or collectively.
- Mechanisms for ensuring all members participate by bringing quality material for reflection in equal measure.
- Reciprocity as the core feature of the working relationship – for example roles of facilitation and administration are shared equally.

Practicalities of Running a Successful Peer Supervision Group

The practicalities of what to take into account when thinking about setting up an effective peer supervision group are discussed including the who, why, what and where of the group. McNally (n.d.) has an excellent, easy-to-read guide for starting a peer supervision group, which can be adapted for an SF group and helpful questions to think about are below.

What Brings Participants Together

Consider what brings the participants together. Some ideas may include:

- Coaches in the same geographical area
- Coaches who all use the same model/framework in their coaching and want to develop their skills with other like-minded practitioners
- Coaches who all work in a similar context, e.g. internal coaches at the same company, a group of external coaches who offer the same type of coaching
- Coaches from the same coaching school who are already in a natural group and want to continue after the end of the course

The Why or Purpose of the Group

"What are the expected outcomes of the group?"

"How will you all know it has been useful?"

Some ideas may include:

- Developing skills in SF coaching
- Reflecting and learning from client work
- Learning to apply coaching skills in new contexts
- Overall personal and professional development of the coach
- Exploring issues of professional conduct and ethical dilemmas

After the purpose of the group is clear, some of the other practicalities can be established.

The Who

"Who will you invite to the group?"

There need to be enough characteristics of the group that are shared so that participants can relate to the topics discussed and to make sense for the group to form, but enough diversity to bring different ideas and points of view to the discussions and make it a rich learning space for all. Valuing diversity and the contributions of different perspectives is key as is mutual respect and curiosity.

Open versus Closed

"Is the group open (members can come and go at any time) or closed (the same group of participants each time)?"

A closed group can be helpful in building the safety and trust in the group, leading to a greater sense of participants' learning. As participants get to know each other over time they may spot themes in what colleagues bring. An open group can bring fresh ideas and may be less likely to become stale and may prevent some of the challenges above of collusion and group think.

"What are the attendance expectations?"

The challenges can be to agree to the expectations of participation – is everyone equally committed to attending each time. Sometimes as a peer group with no fees or supervisor to check attendance, not everyone may attend and attendance expectations need clarifying at the start of the group.

"If the group is small to begin with, can new members join?"

"Who decides whether someone can join –is this by consensus of the group?"

How Many People Should Attend

According to the literature an ideal number varies slightly. Clutterbuck et al. (2016) recommend 6–8; McNicoll (2008) recommends 4–8; and Turner et al. (2018) recommend 5–7.

Sometimes when starting a group, numbers may be smaller as it can take time to build up membership.

The Where

"Where will the group meet?"

"Will it be in person on online?"

The aim is to make the group as easy as possible for people to attend.

Since the pandemic many peer supervision groups have been conducted online so participants can join from anywhere making it convenient for people to attend during their workday. This needs someone willing to host the online meeting space or can be rotated across the members.

If in person, the group needs to decide if there a fixed place to meet (ideally near public transport, centrally located, and easy to find) or whether the venue will rotate with each member taking turns to host. The room needs to be large enough to accommodate the group comfortably but not be so large the group feels lost in the room if less people attend. Good facilities such as restrooms, access to refreshments and enough chairs that are easy to arrange so that every member can see each other are important.

The When

"How often will the group meet?"

"How long will the group meet for?"

Many supervision groups meet on a monthly basis for at least 90 minutes, but the group can decide the frequency and length that works best in their setting.

Co-creating a Well-Functioning Peer Supervision Group

After clarifying the purpose of the group and establishing the group membership and practicalities, the importance of setting up a good psychological contract is key.

Outlined below are some ideas that help to create and maintain the benefits outlined above, and minimise and manage the challenges.

Contracting

A good contracting process that is regularly reviewed is the key to all successful supervision. Having detailed discussions at the outset of the group already minimises the likelihood of problems in the group later as the group process has been co-created by all group members. There is also then a clear mandate about what to do if any challenges are noticed.

Many of the questions in Chapter 11 on group supervision (see pp. 159–177) are all useful here – changing from the supervisor asking the group, to the group asking each other best hopes from and for the group:

- What are our individual best hopes **from** the group?
- What difference are we hoping the group makes for our coaching practice?
- Who will notice when the group goes well (e.g. manager, clients, colleagues)?
- What will they be noticing?
- What are our best hopes **for** the group so it has the highest potential of helping us towards our personal best hopes?
- What else are we hoping our group will be like?
- How would that show up in the ways we are with each other?
- What do we hope to be learning in this group?
- What will each of us be contributing to add value to this group?
- How can we **be** together so that everyone benefits and our time together is constructive and developmental?
- What else do we need to be aware of?

Some of the questions from Chapter 11 on the role of the supervisor (see pp. 159–177) can be adapted as outlined below:

- Suppose there was a video of the group, how would an observer be able to tell this is a peer supervision group rather than supervisor led group?
- From previous experiences of group supervision, what would we like us all to do? What would we hope we don't do?
- What roles do we need in the group and how often will these rotate (e.g. presenter, facilitator, time keeper, coordinator of logistics)?
- What other questions come to mind that we need to discuss?
- How will we deal with challenges within the group?
- How will each of us take responsibility for addressing challenges in the group?
- How will we make sure everyone has a voice in the group?
- What will we do if certain people are always quiet or someone seems to dominate the group?
- How confident are we about taking our own responsibility for learning in the group?
- How often will we review our group?
- How will we review our group?
- How will we let each other know if we need to adjust the group process in any way?

Reviewing the Group

Contracting is not a one-off process, so it is important to also set up a regular review of the group so that any difficulties noticed can be addressed early. Useful SF questions include:

- What has been going well in the group so far?
- What would we like more of, less of or to do differently going forwards?

Content of the Group

At the start of the group appropriate topics for the group can be discussed and then each session an agenda made. Typical standing discussion items may include case presentations, professional challenges; ethical dilemmas; new trends; sharing resources or research alerts.

- What kind of topics will we bring to the group?
- What topics would not be suitable for the group?
- How often will we each present a case?
- How will we organise a rota for presentations?
- Will we also have some informal time at the start or end of the group?

If the group is an SF peer group, it can be helpful to agree that when presenting cases or topics, the questions and suggestions given fit with the SF coaching approach. As outlined in Chapter 11 on group supervision, the SF supervision moves can be useful here (see Chapter 11, pp. 159–177).

Or the group may agree that even if the process is SF, suggestions from any model or framework can be shared to enhance learning and different perspectives.

Reflecting Team

The reflecting team model as outlined in Chapter 11 also lends itself very well to peer supervision groups, and the group can take it in turns to present and rotate the facilitator role.

See Chapter 11, pp. 159–177, for a full description of the reflecting team process and Appendix, pp. 238–247, for the transcript of the reflecting team.

Case Examples

Two case examples are shared below that illustrate a group that went smoothly from the beginning, and another group where there were some challenges and how these were addressed. Learning points from these experiences are offered.

Case Example 1

An experienced coach moved to a new country and reached out to find other English speaking professionals with whom to connect. After initial networking meetings to get to know each other better, one person suggested setting up a peer supervision group. All had shared similar frustrations of feeling isolated in their work as external coaches in private practice and were pleased to connect. After meeting with numerous professionals, a small group of six experienced coaches decided to meet to explore whether they had enough in common to benefit from a peer supervision group. All were English speaking and working in a European country – facing the challenges of working in a system where English was not the majority language and there were numerous challenges of running a business and liaising with other professionals locally.

All used different models in their work, but all had a similar number of years' experience. Sharing the challenges faced by living and working in a foreign country and normalising the frustrations were a big part of the purpose of the group.

The first session involved setting up the structure and ground rules of the group. It was agreed the group would meet for 2 hours over lunch once a month. There would be some informal time to talk over lunch and then the formal peer supervision meeting would start. There would be one case presentation each month. Each member would present a case twice a year and the rota was set up 6 months in advance. Each person would take turns to host and facilitate the meeting – which included arranging the venue for lunch. So that what was discussed in the group was confidential, it was agreed that meeting in a restaurant would only work if there was a private room available, otherwise the facilitator would host in their office meeting room and order lunch. At the start of each meeting, an agenda in addition to the case presentation was discussed and agreed. When presenting cases, the reflecting team model was used where the presenter would ask a question of the group, present the case and then the group members offer observations and reflections. The presenter would then share what had been useful and ask questions of the group if they needed any clarification about the suggestions offered. While everyone was keen to meet, it was agreed that one of the rules for the group to run well was that attendance was expected barring illness or emergency. Dates for the group were set up a year ahead and were the same day and time of the month to make diary planning easy. During summer and Christmas where many would be away, the dates were changed if needed around group members holidays.

Reflections

This group met with the same participants for over 3 years until one member left the country. The group then interviewed and agreed on another member to join and still continue to meet. What helped this group run well was the selection of members at the start, keeping it small and a closed group. This group worked really well as all members were equally experienced in being part of and running groups themselves, so all were happy to take turns to be the facilitator. The group made a big difference to the sense of professional belonging while working in a foreign country and many collaborations and projects came out of the group members' relationships that had been formed.

Case Example 2: Solution Focused Group for Coaches

Prior to the pandemic a peer supervision group for SF practitioners met monthly initiated by one of the graduates of the Academy of Solution Focused Training in Singapore. Due to the pandemic, the group stopped meeting as the group had previously been meeting physically in various locations. There had been several attempts to restart and redesign the peer supervision group over the 11 years the group had been meeting. About a year after the pandemic, one of the authors (Jane) returned to Singapore and having fond memories of attending the group as a participant in the past, offered to take the group online and set it back up. An email was sent to all graduates of the Academy to gauge interest and an initial meeting set up to discuss what people wanted from a group. Following a positive first meeting, dates and times were agreed – monthly over lunchtime via zoom. Everyone wanted a space to meet with other SF practitioners and develop their skills in using the model, agreed to regular case presentations using the SF reflecting team described in Chapter 11 (see pp. 159–177) and to make agenda items on various topics as the need arose. All seemed good. However, it became clear after two to three meetings that no one was volunteering to present or facilitate. As an experienced group supervisor, Jane found this puzzling, as this was a peer group and it was not being addressed. This brought home the interesting challenge in setting up a peer group – by taking on the initiator role and being the zoom host, it was difficult for others not to view her as the supervisor. She suggested another meeting to review progress. The group revisited the ground rules, had discussions about how to make the group feel safer for people to volunteer to present and facilitate. What emerged from the review process was that while the group shared the same model, everyone worked in different settings and were concerned whether what they presented would have any value to others in the group. Would someone doing youth coaching gain from listening to someone working as a health or executive coach? Also many of the group were newly trained, so some wondered if the more experienced members would get value from their presentations. Getting these concerns out in the open was important as members were then able to share that actually hearing about other types of clients that they didn't normally work with would enhance their knowledge and skills, and as the SF process is the same no matter the presenting issue, there is still much to gain from listening to others' presentations. It also emerged that many people did not have experience facilitating in groups and were nervous about trying this for the first time. After this discussion, people felt more comfortable signing up to present and all agreed that if the facilitator needed help at any point they would ask the group. We reviewed the process again 6 months later and all agreed this was working well. The group has so far been meeting for 3 years. A regular group has attended since the beginning. Each 6 months any more trained coaches are invited to attend so there is also refreshing newness to the group.

We decided to have a "closed open" group, i.e., that there were a fixed number of people on the list for the group for each 6-month period and people committed to attending at least 4 out of 6 months sessions. This way there was a continuous core of people attending but allowed for other commitments to be attended to without affecting the overall group, and new members brought a freshness and new ideas to the group.

Reflections

This was a really useful learning experience for Jane as a supervisor about how to step back from this role when in a peer group and let the group discover its way forwards. It was also useful learning that a peer supervision group can take time to get into a rhythm and needs regular reviews to check what is working well and how to adapt to support all member's needs.

Exercise

If you are already in peer group supervision these are some questions that might be helpful to use to review the group:

- What is going well in our group? What else (keep asking the what else question until a rich detailed picture of all the things going well is built up)?

- What might we notice as our group works even better together?
- What questions or ideas from this chapter would we like to bring to the group for more discussion?

If you are not yet in peer group supervision:

- What has inspired you from this chapter?
- How might you take these ideas forwards?

References

Bannink, F. (2015). *Handbook of positive supervision for supervisors, facilitators, and peer groups*. Hogrefe Publishing GmbH.

Bellersen, M., & Kohlmann, I. (2016). *Intervision: Dialogue methods in action learning*. Vakmedianet.

Cambridge Dictionary (n.d.). Peer. In Cambridge Dictionary online. Retrieved 24 January, 2024, from https://dictionary.cambridge.org/dictionary/english/peer

Clutterbuck, D., Whitaker, C., & Lucas, M. (2016). *Coaching supervision: A practical guide for supervisees*. Routledge.

Lippmann, E. (2009). *Intervision, kollegiales coaching professionell gestalten* (2nd edn). Springer.

Martin, P., Milne, D.L., & Reiser, R.P. (2017). Peer supervision: International problems and prospects. *Journal of Advanced Nursing, 74*(5), 998–999. https://doi.org/10.1111/jan.13413

McNicoll, A. (2008 October 22). *Peer supervision – No one knows as much as all of us*. New Zealand Coaching and Mentoring Centre. https://www.coachingmentoring.co.nz/articles/peer-supervision-no-one-knows-much-all-us

McNally, J. (n.d.). *How to start and run a peer supervision group*. Association for Contextual Behavioural Science. https://contextualscience.org/how_to_start_and_run_a_peer_supervision_group_julian_mcnally

Pliopas, A. (2021). Meaning-making encounters: The strength of peer supervision. In J. Birch (Ed) *Coaching supervision groups* (pp. 51–61). Routledge.

Proctor, B. (2008). *Group supervision* (pp. 126–139). Sage Publications.

SolutionsAcademy. (2023). *Coaching Supervision Session 20: Peer Supervision and Intervision*. [Course Presentation]. SolutionsAcademy. https://www.solutionsacademy.com/coach-training/sf-coaching-supervision

Standards Australia. (2011). *HB 332-2011 coaching in organizations*. SAI Global.

Turner, T., Lucas, M., & Whitaker, C. (2018). *Peer supervision in coaching and mentoring: A versatile guide for reflective practice*. Routledge.

Udale, B., & Routt, B. (2021). Linking learning: A peer supervision chain. In J. Birch (Ed) *Coaching supervision groups* (pp. 164–180). Routledge.

13 Team Coaching Supervision

Cristina Mühl and Carlo Perfetto

Introduction

"As yet, there is no one clear model for supervising team coaches. Supervisors tend to adapt to the team context with existing models from supervising one-to-one coaching" (Clutterbuck et al., 2019, e-book, Chapter 23, "Models and methods", para 1). This chapter starts with clarifying what team coaching is and the SF approach to team coaching so that any individual coaching supervisor can familiarise themselves with what it might take to undertake team coaching supervision. We then provide a description of what team coaching supervision is and the difference the SF stance makes to team coaching supervision. We distinguish between team coaching supervision, individual coaching supervision and group supervision. We offer some common topics that team coaching supervision clients might bring and what challenges can arise for the team coaching supervisor. Resources to have available are included for team coaching supervisors to transform those challenges into growth opportunities for the team coaching supervision client.

While this chapter primarily focuses on coaching supervision of team coaches, there may be others who can benefit from what team coaching supervision offers. Examples include trainers, mediators, team leaders, scrum masters, agile coaches and project managers. All engage with teams and groups and may experience challenges similar to those of team coaches, and hence may be interested in the same type of exploration and developmental conversation that team coaching supervision offers to team coaches.

The last sections of the chapter address specific emergent applications of team coaching supervision, namely team coaching supervision with the team in the session.

We encourage the reader to use the section on team coaching and SF team coaching either as a refresher or as a general overview. If the reader is better served to move directly to the potential moves in team coaching supervision or any other section of the chapter, please do so.

DOI: 10.4324/9781003390527-13

What Is Team Coaching and What Is Solution Focused Team Coaching?

Team coaching, as guided by the European Mentoring and Coaching Council (EMCC) and International Coaching Federation (ICF) team coaching frameworks (EMCC Global, 2015b; International Coaching Federation, n.d.a), involves working with a collection of individuals who identify as a team (not a group) to enhance their collective performance and effectiveness. A team is defined by having a common purpose and interrelated tasks to carry out. A group of people all independently working towards a common goal, for example, typists typing individual documents, are not a team. They are not interdependent on one another to accomplish the desired results.

In the first chapters of our book, we emphasised the SF approach's recognition of multiple perspectives and truths in individual supervision. This concept encourages individuals to value diverse viewpoints, leading to richer insights and outcomes. Similarly, in team coaching supervision, SF team coaches are encouraged to apply this principle. This is in line with the ICF team coaching competency framework which states that the team coach "fosters expression of individual team members and the collective team's feelings, perceptions, concerns, beliefs, hopes, and suggestions" (International Coaching Federation, n.d.a).

This approach enables teams to harness the diversity of perspectives and generate greater value in their coaching journey.

From an SF stance, there are some key aspects of the team coaching process that will be useful to keep in mind in the supervision space (Dierolf et al., 2023, pp. 8–11):

- *Pluralism – differences of view*: As team coaches, we are always dealing with multiple perspectives and truths. Each team member has their own truth – the manager will have theirs, as will other stakeholders. All are true, but none are THE TRUTH.
- *Team is at the centre*: In SF team coaching, the team coach will hold the assumption that every case is different, every team is different and that there are no predefined qualities of a high-performing or dysfunctional team. The desired outcomes from the team coaching are not defined by a diagnostic instrument, but by the team itself.
- *Flux – differences of state*: In our view, individual and team identities are connected to the stories that are being told about the individual or the team by the individual themselves or by others. We strive to invite our clients to "tell their stories in ways that make them stronger" (Wingard & Lester, 2001).

Team coaching is co-created: We believe that a coaching process always changes both the coach and the client(s). The relevant system consists of all stakeholders including the coach.

Opening space – expanding choice: SF team coaches will try to be curious and aware that their own assumptions are just that: assumptions and not truths. Of course, we are human and there is no way to be human and not have assumptions – you can't live questioning your assumptions that the floor will hold, and a new day will be there tomorrow, for example. The difference is that we try not to turn our assumptions into truth.

Opening space for enlivened possibilities: SF team coaches invite clients to talk about what they are wanting rather than what they are not wanting. They focus on what is already going in the right direction, thereby opening space for more possibility: the team coaching is more about describing the preferred future than about analysing and classifying the past.

Enacting an ethics of caring and privileging restorative justice: The team coach is the advocate for collaboration of the team, not the advocate of any individual team member. This is relevant, even when there are serious accusations or difficulties that happened in the team.

Team coaching requires the proficient use of several modalities by the team coach. The team coach needs coaching skills, facilitation skills, conflict management skills, training skills and so on. These skills are not something you can learn by reading a book or in a theoretical way. You can only develop them through practice, and you can improve by Deliberate Practice and Reflective Practice (which are outlined in Chapters 8 and 9 in more detail). There is no one way to coach or one way to facilitate – every coach and team coach develops their own style. Everyone struggles with different situations: one team coach might have trouble helping a team come to a clear goal, the other might shy away from mentioning potential conflicts. Therefore, after initial training, a way to develop team coaching capability is by regularly working with a team coaching supervisor.

We hope this short overview provides sufficient insight into the world of team coaching to set the basis for moving the focus to team coaching supervision. More on team coaching can be found in *Solution Focused Team Coaching* (Dierolf et al., 2023).

What Is Team Coaching Supervision?

In this section we will look at why team coaches seek supervision, what happens in team coaching supervision, what the role of the supervisor could be and what the differences between team coaching supervision and individual supervision are.

Team coaches acknowledge that supervision is vital. They draw on a range of methods to support themselves, which includes one-to-one, group and peer supervision. What team coaches are seeking and value is a safe place to stand back from the client team to identify the patterns and themes that emerge. They want to explore from outside the system what may be happening both within the team and for themselves, and how to stay with the unpredictability of what arises. Supervision also provides the platform for the coach to identify new ways to take the team forward.

(Bachkirova et al., 2021, pp. 254–263)

Passmore in "A Manifesto for Supervision" presents a summary of statistical results of different surveys exploring supervision (Hawkins et al., 2019). One of these surveys from 2017, with 2,791 participants from a total of 45 European countries, of which nearly 1,000 were from the UK, found lower levels of engagement with supervision. Thirty-four per cent said they did not engage in supervision, and of more than 2,000 responses, 35.3% said they expected to get reflective practice for free, with a further 17.5% expecting it to cost less than 50 Euros per hour. At the same time, the result of a research study undertaken by Palmer in 2017, notes "respondents also reported that supervision enhanced coaching performance and their wellbeing, the latter being an under-researched area of the benefits of supervision" (Palmer, 2017).

Unfortunately, there are no comparable statistics around team coaching supervision. A limited study around "Ethical Dilemmas in Team Coaching" was conducted by Cristina Mühl in 2023 and 24% of respondents (all team coaches) mentioned that they use supervision to explore ethical dilemmas. Another 24% use peer conversations to explore ethical dilemmas (Mühl, 2023).

"From a Solution Focused perspective, clinical supervision can be defined as facilitating the development of competent professionals, enhancing the professional's knowledge and skills, and assisting them in serving their customers" (Thomas, 2013, p. 240). This is equally valid for team coaching supervision. Team coaching supervision is a facilitated conversation around the elements mentioned above with the desire to support the development of professional team coaches and to enhance the work they do with their team coaching clients.

Team coaching supervision is not only a method for quality assurance but can serve as a restorative function, namely to help a team coach process any negative experiences or stressors that occur during team coaching. Restorative learning and receiving of support are optimised when supervision takes place with a team coaching supervisor who clearly communicates their respect for the resourcefulness and capability of the team coach.

Frank Thomas (2013) proposes a variety of roles for supervisors, namely, acting as a "guru", "gatekeeper" and/or "guide". These roles are outlined in more detail in Chapter 5, see pp. 59–75. Team coaches seem to be better served by a mix of these roles depending also on the expertise of the team coach. In our experience, many inexperienced team coaches look for guidance and clarification during their team coaching supervision, while more experienced team coaches engaging in supervision are looking for a partner to further their practice and thinking. Rather than adopting a rigid process, team coaching supervision needs to be sufficiently flexible to suit the developmental needs of each team coach.

Sundman (Thomas 2013, pp. 239–250) raises yet another role for the supervisor which arises in long-term supervision. Sundman proposes that the role is more like that of a consultant with a focus on expansion of the practitioner's repertoire. In relation to team coaching supervision, adopting such a consultation offers the team coach support to expand their capability to manage the complexities that arise in team coaching, complexities which are different from those arising in individual coaching.

The purposes of team coaching supervision include, but are not limited to reflection on past engagements, identifying what went well, figuring out what could go better, exploring best hopes/desired outcomes and possibilities for interactions in any given team coaching engagement. Team coaching supervision can also be used as a preparation for a team coaching engagement. Here the team coach shares their plans with the team coaching supervisor, asks for advice, brainstorms together, and is supported to go into the next engagement prepared mentally, emotionally and organisationally.

Differences and Similarities Between Team Coaching Supervision and Individual and Group Coaching Supervision

In order to sharpen the awareness of what team coaching supervision requires, we offer some differences and similarities between team coaching supervision and individual coaching supervision and between team coaching supervision and group coaching supervision.

Differences and Similarities Between Team Coaching Supervision and Individual Coaching Supervision

The work of a team coach is often more complex than individual coaching, as there are several other elements to take into account when contracting all the way through to the facilitation of the team coaching workshops. It is common for team coaching sessions to be referred to as "workshops": which can lead to confusion with skills training. However, we use the term "workshops" in this chapter as it is part of the regular terminology of team coaches.

In response to the added complexity, the role of the team coaching supervisor is enhanced to include exploring with the team coach not only the case/content/situation, but also to invite the team coach to reflect upon the co-creation of relationships, process and knowledge.

Questions that might be used to explore facilitation might include:

- What were your best hopes around setting up the session in that way?
- What is important for you in the facilitation?
- What is the role of facilitation in the process from your perspective?
- How would you like the team to perceive the session?

As you might have noticed from the way SF team coaching supervision is defined, there are many similarities with individual SF coaching supervision. That is because the stance of an SF supervisor remains the same. It is grounded in the tenets of pragmatism, tentativeness, curiosity and respect (for more details, see Chapter 3, pp. 27–42). The difference between individual and team coaching supervision resides more in the topics and the needs of the supervision client, than in the stance of the team coaching supervisor.

Team Coaching Supervision and Group Coaching Supervision

When we talk about team coaching supervision, the most common scenario is one team coach attending an individual supervision session with a team coaching supervisor. Team coaches can however also be supervised in a group.

Group coaching supervision, when the group consists of individual coaches primarily focuses on individual coaching skills, techniques and approaches used by each coach in the group. It aims to help coaches refine their coaching abilities, explore coaching methodologies and address any challenges they encounter in their coaching practice.

When supervising team coaches in group coaching supervision, the extent of exploration is different as it extends beyond individual coaching skills to include the co-creation of relationships, the process of team coaching and the relevant knowledge.

It is important therefore that coaching supervisors are aware of the specific needs of team coaches, and if supervising team coaches in a group make sure the focus extends to the exploration of factors that are relevant to team coaches. It is also important that they are aware of managing the challenges that can present when supervising in a group setting (see Chapter 11 for more details on group coaching supervision).

What Is Solution Focused Team Coaching Supervision?

The SF approach assumes that coaching supervisors do not position themselves above the coaching supervision client. The SF approach holds the foundational assumption that the coaching supervision client has resources and expertise to generate improvements for their team coaching engagements. The team coaching supervisor is viewed as positioned at the intersection of the co-creation of relationships, process and knowledge and as opening a conversational space for the team coach to reflect on what is happening in their practice and how they want to show up as a team coach (as depicted in Figure 13.1).

As illustrated above, team coaching supervision will mostly address:

- the co-creation of relationships – with the team or teams that the team coach is engaging with,
- the process – either the overall team coaching process or the process within a team coaching workshop and
- the knowledge – be it specific team coaching knowledge or allied knowledge such as facilitation.

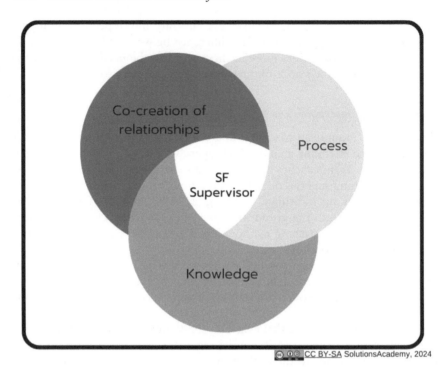

Figure 13.1 An integrated view of team coaching supervision (Image by Cristina Muhl)

SF supervision brings a focus of keeping things simple (despite the complexities of working with teams) and co-creating the conversation in the team coaching supervision sessions that allows space for the team coach to explore what needs to happen in the team coaching sessions, and also to define the best way in which the team coaching supervisor can support them.

Here follow some assumptions around team coaching and team coaching supervision that we feel need to be addressed in order to create a better picture of what happens in an SF team coaching supervision session in line with the structure proposed above (co-creation of relationships, process and knowledge):

The co-creation lens. In some forms of team coaching supervision, there is the assumption that the team needs to be evaluated and assessed by the team coaching supervisor and the team coach. In contrast, SF team coaching supervisors hold the assumption that the team coach sits at the centre of the team coaching supervision, assessment of the team is likely to be counter-productive due to encouraging rigidity and thinking in labels that describe fixed states. SF supervision holds the focus on exploring the co-creation of a flexible, adaptive web of relationships amongst the team coach and the team members, which best serves the desired outcome of the team.

In the SF approach, there is a deliberate choice to centre the discussion on the supervision client – the team coach in this case, rather than on the clients of the team coaching supervision client – the team being coached.

"One of the important practices in SF supervision is to challenge conclusions about people and guide conversations toward possibility" (Thomas, 2013, pp. 20–21). During team coaching supervision sessions, the primary emphasis is on the team coach's experience, reflections and insights. The SF team coaching supervisor focuses the conversation on inviting a rich description from the team coaching supervision client about how they are approaching the team coaching process, coping with challenges and opportunities and utilising Solution Focused techniques. In this way, the team coach engages in self-reflection and learning, which expands their awareness of and confidence in their team coaching style, strategies and the benefits of their contributions to the results accomplished by the team via team coaching.

SF team coaching supervision holds the perspective of "supervisor-and-team-coach-and-their-team-as-a-system", while the traditional view of team coaching supervision is "team-coach-and-their-team-as-system" (Dierolf et al., 2023). This difference in perspective is illustrated in Figures 13.2 and 13.3:

The SF team coaching supervisor opens a space for the team coaching supervision client to clarify their perspective, beliefs and assumptions.

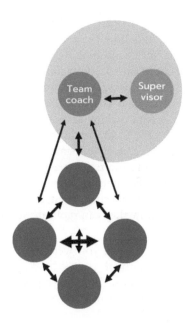

Figure 13.2 Solution Focused team coaching puts the team coach at the centre of the conversation (Image by Kirsten Dierolf)

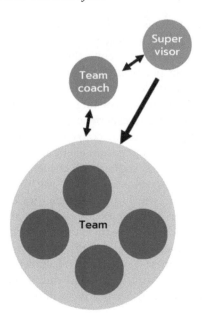

Figure 13.3 Traditional team coaching supervision model where the team coach and the supervisor engage in analysing the team (Image by Kirsten Dierolf)

This supports the team coach to gain insight into their own thoughts and decision-making processes, and how these influence their coaching interactions with the team. The team coaching supervision conversation aims to identify the strengths of the team coaching supervision client and their work with the team thus far. By recognising what is working well, together the team coaching supervisor and the team coaching supervision client can build on these strengths for future team coaching sessions.

Another contribution by the team coaching supervisor is to provide feedback on the team coach's coaching style, communication and strategies. This feedback is intended to support the team coach's ongoing development and enhance their effectiveness in facilitating positive change with the team. The feedback can involve asking SF questions that prompt the coach to explore what has been effective and how they can replicate success, such as:

- When were some moments when you were at your best with this team? What were you contributing then?
- What are you noticing about how the team responds well in relation to who you are being as a team coach? How can you amplify those aspects in your future interactions?
- Let's suppose you find just the way to be the best team coach for this team given their desired outcome, what might the team notice about you?

- Imagine for a moment that you've perfectly aligned your coaching approach with the team's desired outcomes. What subtle shifts might the team members start recognising in your presence and interactions? How would they describe the impact on their collaboration and progress?

By avoiding discussions about the supervision client's clients (the team being coached), the focus remains squarely on the team coach. This intentional choice aims to create a space where the coach can explore and deepen their understanding without being distracted by external factors. This approach encourages the team coach to take ownership and accountability for their coaching practice. It emphasises the coach's agency in driving positive change within the team and helps them feel more empowered in their role.

The process lens: There is the assumption that team coaching requires the management of both complex and complicated processes and hence requires the team coach to review appropriate tools and techniques in team coaching supervision. SF team coaching supervisors view is that the degree of complexity is set by what serves the team coaching client well, with a leaning towards simplifying and demystifying rather than complicating the team coaching process.

What does this mean for team coaching supervision? The perspective adopted in SF team coaching supervision is characterised by:

1 *Simplicity and co-creation:* Rather than viewing team coaching as an overly complex endeavour, the approach encourages a belief that team coaching can be approached in a straightforward manner, focusing on what is practical and effective. Reflecting on the team coaching process in its totality and not overcomplicating things by too much analysis of details, is encouraged. In some ways this is a paradox as the SF approach is known for encouraging richly detailed descriptions, but usually of best hopes and of possibilities, rather than of what is not working, or is no longer desired.

2 *Focus on next steps:* The SF approach encourages a focus on practical solutions and tangible outcomes. By not perceiving team coaching as overly complex, the emphasis shifts towards identifying straightforward and actionable steps that can lead to positive changes for the team. This allows the team coach to take away from their team coaching supervision a clear path for engaging in future sessions with the teams they are coaching.

3 *Trust in the expertise of the team coach:* The SF team coaching supervisor evokes and supports the ability of the team coaching supervision client to navigate their team coaching sessions without being overwhelmed or disempowered by deficit-thinking, anticipating complications and assuming they lack the capability to undertake the job they contracted to do. The team coaching supervision client is supported in identifying when they may require additional resourcing, but not to assume incompetence, but rather to think something like "I am not yet as resourced as I need to be to respond to what I am now experiencing with this team. I have a plan of how to resource myself even more".

4 *Encouragement of a growth-oriented mindset:* An SF perspective often encourages a positive mindset, seeing challenges as opportunities for growth rather than as insurmountable obstacles. By not characterising team coaching as excessively complex, the focus is on the positive aspects and potential solutions both in the supervision and the team coaching process.

5 *Create a learning environment:* Viewing team coaching as not overwhelming fosters an environment where both team coaches and their team coaching supervisors are more open to learning, adaptation and continuous improvement. It suggests an approach that is agile and responsive to the evolving needs of all involved in the team coaching.

6 *Collaboration:* When team coaching is not seen as overwhelmingly or overly complicated, a collaborative and inclusive atmosphere is promoted. Team members, team coaches and the team coaching supervisor are more likely to engage in open communication and work together towards shared goals. It also creates the potential for a team coaching supervision session with the team in the room, where all parties are viewed as being able to add value.

The knowledge lens: There is the assumption that a team coach should be equipped with theories and concepts, for example, in group dynamics, developmental stages of teams, and how to manage resistance. SF team coaching supervision invites team coaches to explore how to optimise the resources and expertise that they, and the team, already have, before assuming that there is a lack of knowledge which requires introducing more theories and concepts. This principle in SF team coaching emphasises a deliberate shift away from external analysis or diagnostic attempts to noticing and describing the interactions of the team. The focus is on exploring and building solutions collaboratively, using already existing knowledge. We can recount several supervision sessions where the team coach came in with notes and ideas around the reasons why the team that they were engaging with acted and reacted in a certain situation, and what that might infer about the team. As SF supervisors we felt it was appropriate to raise the question "Have you considered sharing these thoughts with the team to gather their ideas and comments?" Instead of using the team coaching supervision session as a time to create a spider-web of assumptions about the team and its functioning, the team coaching supervisor invites the team coaching supervision client to move towards reflecting on their noticings and responses to the team. Instead of trying to understand the underlying issues from an external perspective, the SF team coaching supervisor engages with the team coaching supervision client in ways that support them to envision and work towards a desired future state by collaborating with the team. In doing so, the SF team coaching supervisor acknowledges the expertise of the team coach and the team itself, trusting that those involved in the team coaching process have the knowledge and resources necessary to generate the desired outcomes.

Possible Moves for Solution Focused Team Coaching Supervision

Providing a step-by-step process for team coaching supervision that would fit all situations is clearly unrealistic. Team coaching comes in different shapes and interactions, so constructing a model that applies every time will result in a rigid way of approaching team coaching supervision. Earlier we mentioned the concept of "flux" and that in an SF approach, we regard "every interaction as mutual influence" with potential for multidirectional influence (Gosnell et al., 2017).

As SF team coaching supervisors, we can envision team coaching supervision as engaging in a set of moves that are aligned with the SF gallery which forms the basic structure for any coaching intervention in both individual coaching and team coaching. This framework can support the team coach in designing and managing a team coaching intervention that respects the basic pillars of the SF approach mentioned at the beginning of this chapter: flow, uniqueness of each intervention, pluralism of views, keeping the team at the centre, co-creation of the intervention, awareness of the assumptions and future orientation. On this basis, the SF gallery can also be usefully considered as a framework for team coaching supervision. These moves are designed to support the team coaching supervision client to explore the three elements of co-creation of relationships, process and knowledge. Chapter 4 presents the gallery in detail (see Figure 4.1). Below we explain how it can be used for team coaching supervision and provide some ideas of what questions can be used.

Ticket office

Defining the scope and purpose of the team coaching supervision conversation and how it will relate to the further development of the team coach's professional identity and ability to undertake their work in alignment with professional team coaching standards.

Some examples of questions that a team coaching supervisor might bring in the ticket office:

- "What part of your work would you like to reflect on today?" "What would you like to be different going forward in relation to this?"
- "Let's explore together the specific areas you'd like to focus on during our team coaching supervision session. What aspects of your professional identity and practice are you keen to develop further?"
- "Considering the purpose or our conversation today, what outcomes would you like to achieve in terms of aligning your work with professional team coaching standards?"

Preferred future: Co-creating a detailed description of the team coaching supervision client being at their best, and what that indicates for the co-creating of relationships with the team, the team coaching process, and the use of their existing knowledge.

Possible questions to be used:

- "If you would enter the next workshop at your best version as a team coach, what would the team notice? How would you respond to their reactions?"

- "As you envision yourself at your best in your team coaching practice, what would that look like in terms of your relationship with the team members?"

Successful past/resources: Questions here can explore past successes when working with teams. Even if the team coach is new to team coaching, each team coach is also a coach. That implies that they have plenty of resources from their individual coaching practice that can be also be activated and explored to see how they can be used in the team coaching process.

For the team coaching accreditation, both ICF and EMCC require coaches to hold an individual coaching credential. That implies that any team coach has gone through an accreditation process that requires understanding the individual core competencies and implementing those in the practice. Those competencies are relevant also in the work that a team coach does and the supervisor can support the team coach in reflecting upon them and identifying what might be useful to re-use also in team coaching.

Several questions can be used such as:

- Can you recall a specific instance where you faced a similar challenge to what you're encountering now in your team coaching practice? How did you navigate that situation successfully, and how might you apply those lessons learned to your current context?
- Reflecting on your past experiences working with different teams, what specific strategies or interventions have consistently led to breakthrough moments or positive shifts in team dynamics?
- In your previous team coaching engagements, what feedback or testimonials have you received from team members or stakeholders regarding the impact of your coaching? How can you leverage these past successes to inform and inspire your current approach?
- "When have you been at a similar stage with an individual client? What was useful back then?"
- "When you started your individual coaching practice, what was useful?"
- "Reflecting on your past experiences as a coach, what specific strengths or strategies have consistently contributed to successful outcomes in your individual coaching practice?"

Gift shop: Here, the analogy is that having spent some time on a visit with the team coaching supervisor, the team coaching supervision client is looking to take away one or more souvenirs that can remind them of what they generated as possibilities. Questions include:

- "What have you learned so far, from your reflections on this team and your interactions with it?"
- "What do you need to feel more confident in working with this team?"
- "What are some steps forward that emerge from this conversation?"
- "What might you want to do to further prepare yourself for the next time you engage with this team?"

There is another layer of the team coaching supervision conversation that needs to be addressed and that includes the following elements:

- *Progress*: To what degree the team coaching supervision session is moving towards the desired outcome and the best hopes of the team coaching supervision client.
- *Relationship*: The influence that the team coaching supervision conversation has on both the team coaching supervisor and the team coaching supervision client. Specific attention is paid to anything that needs to be addressed to enhance their collaboration.
- *Purpose*: As the team coaching supervision process may take place over a period of time such as months, and even years, the purpose of the team coaching supervision needs to be revisited regularly.

Common Topics in Team Coaching Supervision

Team coaching is an emerging profession and the set of core competencies from EMCC (EMCC Global, 2015a), AC (Association for Coaching, n.d.) and ICF (International Coach Federation, n.d.a) has brought the opportunity to reflect upon the type of work that a team coach is doing. In that context it might be considered that the role of a team coaching supervisor will be about supporting the team coach to reflect upon the team development modalities that they employ and how they clarify these with the stakeholders, team leader and team.

In our experience, topics brought to team coaching supervision by team coaches include:

- contracting – contracting with the sponsor that differs from contracting with the team,
- contracting team coaching services when the team is in need of something else,
- contracting when the buyer of team coaching doesn't have a clear understanding of team coaching,
- reflecting on their ongoing learning,
- challenges faced in the coaching process and
- responding to the evolving needs of the teams they work with.

Table 13.1 shows some common challenges that team coaches might bring into team coaching supervision and some possible responses by team coaching supervisors:

These topics provide a broad overview, and the team coaching supervisor should expect the unexpected and welcome the creativity and opportunity that supporting a team coaching supervision client to develop a response to the issue they face brings.

Table 13.1 Common Challenges Faced by Team Coaches and Possible Responses from the Team Coaching Supervisor

Challenge	Description	Possible Response/Solution from the Supervisor
Co-creation of the relationship		
Goal setting	Discussing the team's goals and objectives, and how well they align with the organisational vision	Exploring ways to set realistic and achievable goals that motivate and inspire the team, while also taking into account the organisation's vision, mission and results
Offering observations to the team	Discussing the process of providing feedback to the team as a whole, as well as to individual team members	Exploring how to create a constructive feedback loop that promotes learning and improvement
Adapting to change	Addressing how the team coaching approach can adapt to changes within the team or the broader organisational context	Discussing strategies for maintaining flexibility and resilience in the team coaching process
Perception that the team coach will "fix" everything	Addressing the perception by the team that the team coaching process will resolve everything, that the change will happen during the team coaching sessions and that the team coach will be the messenger to the organisation on behalf of the team	Reflection on the co-creation of the relationship and on the role that the team coach wants to contract with the team Clarifying the responsibilities of the team and each of its members to take actions to initiate and maintain the desired improvements outside of the team coaching sessions
Process		
Coaching strategies	Reflecting on the effectiveness of coaching strategies employed during team sessions	Offering feedback on specific interventions and exploring alternative approaches
Integration with organisational goals	Discussing how team coaching aligns with organisational goals and contributes to broader strategic objectives	Exploring ways to strengthen the integration of team coaching within the organisational context
Misaligned goals between the sponsors (leadership/HR) and the team	Leadership uses team coaching to bring their employees into line with what leadership wants, without listening to what the team wants and/or needs	Facilitating the reflection around the process that can create the space for the different perceptions to be expressed

(*Continued*)

Table 13.1 (Continued)

Challenge	Description	Possible Response/Solution from the Supervisor
Individual team member development	Addressing individual team members' needs for growth and development	Discussing team coaching approaches that support the personal and professional development of team members
		How to expand the contract to offer individual coaching as well as team coaching. Attending to the ethical dilemmas that may arise if the team coach is also the coach offering the individual coaching
Utilising strengths	Discussing how to identify and leverage the strengths of individual team members and the team as a whole	Exploring strategies to notice and then build on what is already working well
Reflecting on successes	Celebrating successes and positive outcomes achieved through team coaching	Reflecting on what contributed to success and identifying factors that can be replicated in future coaching sessions
Ethical dilemmas	Addressing ethical considerations and dilemmas that may arise during team coaching	Discussing ways to notice and navigate ethical challenges, while maintaining alignment with Codes of Ethics, and professional coaching standards
Knowledge		
Handling difficult conversations	Exploring challenges related to addressing conflicts or difficult conversations within the team	Discussing approaches to facilitate constructive dialogue and reaching resolution. "Good enough/we can live with this" vs "Ideal/perfect" resolutions
Team coaching tools and techniques	Reviewing and discussing the application of specific team coaching tools and techniques	Exploring new tools or adapting existing ones based on the unique needs of the team coach and /or the team
Continuous learning and professional development	Exploring opportunities for the team coach's own continuous learning and professional development	Discussing relevant literature, training or resources that can enhance team coaching skills
		Encouraging belonging to professional organisations and/or team coaching communities of practice

Challenges for the Team Coaching Supervisor

We have selected below three of the often mentioned challenges by team coaching supervisors. They pose a particular challenge as they sit at the border of how team coaching supervision is perceived:

1 Supervisor or advisor/teacher for the team coach
2 Supervisor and supervision client coming from the different method/ approach
3 Bringing "self" of the supervisor in the supervision process

For each of these three challenges we have included some suggestions/ ideas on how to approach them.

Generally, the team coaching supervisor would be sitting at the intersection between co-creation of relationships, process and knowledge:

- *Co-creation of relationships*: The supervisor can shift the focus from the specific topic to the bigger picture. Create a moment to reflect on what type of team coach they want to be, how they want to be seen by the team as team coach, and how that would be supported by the way the co-construction will happen in the workshop. In this way the team coach will learn how to look at the forest instead of watching the trees.
- *Process*: The SF supervisor can let the team coach reflect on their idea of "being the best team coach they want to be in that situation", what difference this can make and who would be noticing that. It will allow for a change of stance and open up possibilities.
- *Knowledge*: Instead of jumping in with a solution, the supervisor can encourage the team coach to do some internal research. The supervisor can ask questions that get them thinking deeply about their own strategies and beliefs. It can be surprising how many ideas the team coach can come up with if the supervisor trusts their ability to reflect.

Talking about "using self" in supervision means that we can also bring some thoughts into the conversation with the desire of supporting the supervision process, which means offering constructive feedback and input to enhance the ideas generated by the team coach

A summary of challenges and possible responses is provided in Table 13.2.

Note that at the time of publishing, neither EMCC nor ICF require a team coaching supervisor to be a team coach or have specific team coaching knowledge or experience. It can be argued that the team coaching experience of a supervisor might make a difference in the team coaching supervision process, but currently there are no studies to support that. This also correlated with the conversation around bringing "self" as a team coach in the team coaching supervision process. As SF practitioners, we would leave that up to the coaching supervision client as we believe in the expertise of the team coach and their best hopes from the coaching supervision session.

Table 13.2 Challenges Faced by the Team Coaching Supervisor and Possible Responses from the Supervisor

Challenge	Description	Possible Response/Solution for the Supervisor
Supervisor or advisor/ teacher?	Team coach expecting advice from the team coaching supervisor on how to contract/design the team coaching process	Reflection on the difference it would make if the team coaching supervisor will step into the role of advisor; offer reflection on the team coach's professional values
	The implications of the term supervisor might signal that the team coaching supervisor will take the stance of guru and teach the team coach how to do things	Explore the role of supervision as conversations with restorative, quality assurance and educational functions
		Encourage the team coach to reflect upon the knowledge accumulated from experience, training, peer conversations
		As the role of a supervisor implies also providing input that might support the supervision process, the supervisor might agree upon the type of knowledge the supervision client might want to explore together with the supervisor
Different philosophical method/ approach	The team coaching supervision client having a different philosophical approach than the team coaching supervisor	Collaborating to create a joint language would be the first step in the supervision session
		Several other ideas covered in Chapter 7 of this book on coaching supervision with clients using different models are also relevant in the case of team coaching supervision (see Chapter 7 for more details)
Using "self" in the supervision	Expectation that the supervisor will bring their own knowledge, experience in the supervision and that means that the supervisor should be a team coach also	Collaborate with the supervision client from the contracting stage to understand what they are expecting and what they are searching for in the supervision space

Evolving Practice – Supervision With the Team Present

As SF supervisors are mainly interested in the co-construction between the team coach and the team, supervising the team and the team coach together is an obvious idea. In our age of online team coaching, it is no longer logistically as difficult to work with all stakeholders. Our diagram of co-creation of relationships, process and knowledge is a helpful guide.

The team coaching supervisor can join a team coaching session somewhere in the middle of a team coaching process and offer a retrospective by asking questions like:

Co-creation of the Relationship

- "What has been going well in your collaboration?"
- "What has everyone contributed so far that has added value– the team members, the team leader, the team coach?"
- "What are some things that everyone could do to help make it even better?"

Process

- "On a scale of 1–10, where 10 is your team coaching process is very fitting, where are you now?"
- "What processes are already working well?"
- "What can be improved? Which processes are not yet working as well as they could?"
- "How can everyone contribute to improving it?"

Knowledge

- "What knowledge are you drawing on that is taking you forward?"
- "What knowledge do you have that you have not yet drawn upon?"
- "What collective intelligence is adding most to your ability to create progress?"

Reflections

At the end of this exploration of SF team coaching supervision, we would invite you to reflect with a couple of questions:

- How do you perceive team coaching supervision compared to individual supervision?
- What opportunities might open up once you explore the subject of team coaching and team coaching supervision?
- What strengths do you already have that would support you as a supervisor of team coaches?

- What is your stance about using self as a team coach in team coaching supervision? Do you believe you need experience and expertise as a team coach to be able to support your supervision clients within team coaching supervision?

References

Association for Coaching. (n.d.). *Coaching Competency Framework.* Retrieved from https://cdn.ymaws.com/www.associationforcoaching.com/resource/resmgr/Accreditation/Accred_General/Coaching_Competency_Framewor.pdf

Bachkirova, T., Jackson, P., & Clutterbuck, D. (2021). *Coaching and mentoring supervision: Theory and practice (2nd Ed).* Open University Press.

Clutterbuck, D., Gannon, J., Hayes, S., Iordanou, I., Lowe, K., & MacKie, D. (Eds.). (2019). *The practitioner's handbook of team coaching.* Routledge.

Dierolf, K., Mühl, C., Perfetto, C., & Szaniawski, R. (2023). *Solution focused team coaching.* Routledge.

EMCC Global. (2015a). *EMCC Global Competence Framework V2.* Retrieved from https://www.emccglobal.org/leadership-development/competences/

EMCC Global. (2015b). *EMCC Global Team Coaching Assessment and Accreditation Framework.* Retrieved from https://www.emccglobal.org/accreditation/tcqa/

Gosnell, F., McKergow, M., Moore, B., Mudry, T., & Tomm, K. (2017). A Galveston declaration. *Journal of Systemic Therapies, 36*(3), 20–26. Retrieved from https://galvestondeclaration.org/

Hawkins, P., Turner, E., & Passmore, J. (2019). *The manifesto for supervision.* Henley Business School and The Association for Coaching.

International Coaching Federation. (n.d.a). *Team Coaching Competencies.* International Coaching Federation. https://coachingfederation.org/team-coaching-competencies

International Coaching Federation. (n.d.b). *Core Competencies.* International Coaching Federation. https://coachingfederation.org/credentials-and-standards/core-competencies

Mühl, C. (2023, June 10). Ethical dilemmas in team coaching. *EMCC global conference.* Prague.

Palmer, S. (2017) Beyond the coaching and therapeutic relationship: the supervisee-supervisor relationship. Keynote given on 15 September at the 7th International Congress of Coaching Psychology, 2017, Aalborg University, Aalborg, Denmark.

Thomas, F.N., (2013). *Solution-focused supervision: A resource-oriented approach to developing clinical expertise.* Springer.

Wingard, B., & Lester, J. (2001). *Telling our stories in ways that make us stronger.* Dulwich Centre Publications.

14 Common Topics Arising in Coaching Supervision

Debbie Hogan, Sukanya Wignaraja and Jane Tuomola

Introduction

In coaching supervision, there are an array of common topics and themes that are presented as challenges for the coaching supervision client. Whether they relate to individual, group, peer or team coaching supervision, addressing these challenging topics in coaching supervision often requires careful reflection and a collaborative and supportive approach, which fits well with Solution Focused (SF) coaching supervision. The coaching supervisor must create a safe and non-judgemental space for coaching supervision clients to explore difficult issues, share experiences and seek guidance in navigating complex situations effectively. The focus of coaching supervision centres around the coaching supervision client's practice, with the aim of learning from this experience through a process of critical reflection (Passmore & McGoldrick, 2009).

While some topics might be unique to certain areas of coaching supervision (e.g. individual versus team coaching supervision), many of these topics are common across the spectrum of coaching supervision. This chapter reviews some of the common topics encountered by coaching supervisors, clustered under the four main functions of coaching supervision, namely, restorative/supportive, personal/professional development, ethics/quality assurance and managerial/commercial that were discussed in Chapter 2. Common topics addressed in the literature are also included to highlight the range of what coaching supervision clients bring to the coaching supervision space.

We bring together all the learnings from across the book, offering some suggestions as to how the coaching supervisor can support the coaching supervision client using SF questions and moves to deal with these topics. As well as drawing on transcripts from earlier in the book where some of these topics are illustrated, additional examples are shared. The coaching supervisor is invited to apply these ideas to their own work via questions and activities for reflection and action.

Background

The International Coaching Federation (ICF) conducted a study titled *Global Coaching Supervision: Study of the Perceptions and Practices Around the World* (McAnally et al., 2020). Data was analysed from 1280 coaches across the globe

DOI: 10.4324/9781003390527-14

from 72 countries, across the continents of Africa, Asia, Australia, Europe and North and South America. The study was conducted to learn more about a broad range of issues brought to coaching supervision, the current state of practice and perceptions of coaches who work with a coaching supervisor.

The two most common topics raised by coaching supervision clients in both individual and group coaching supervision were found to be client-related issues, challenges and situations, and personal-related issues, challenges and situations.

Coaching supervision clients reported that the most helpful coaching supervisor contribution was when their coaching supervisor offered their own perspective, ideas, advice and/or experience and offered more direct constructive developmental feedback during coaching supervision sessions. The study also revealed that the most helpful coaching supervisor behaviours were those which helped the coaching supervision client to improve their coaching skills and their own positive self-regard.

Hawkins et al. (2019) reported that the top concerns brought to coaching supervision are anxiety and fear of shame and judgement and challenges with contracting. Passmore (2009) mentions challenging client cases and ethical dilemmas as top concerns raised by coaching supervision clients.

Clutterbuck et al. (2016) list a number of common topics and areas that a coaching supervision client could consider bringing to coaching supervision. They list topics concerned with formative aspects of coaching supervision (developing your repertoire as a coach), normative issues (conflicts or ethical dilemmas, restorative issues (coaching has had an impact on you personally) and performative issues (your whole person and continuing journey of self-discovery). They suggest different strategies of preparing for coaching supervision that relate to a client issue such as reviewing something that has already occurred through case notes or recordings, analysing critical incidents, reviewing client feedback or planning ahead for something that has yet to happen. Other topics to bring to coaching supervision could be themes noticed across your coaching practice as a whole, a personal issue, focusing on education content such as a theoretical concept to develop more understanding or business development concerns.

They also created four categories of broad themes to help prompt discussion when a coaching supervision client has no topic. These include confidentiality, for example, handling information when working with multiple stakeholders, boundaries, for example, straying from coaching to other modalities, conflicts of interest, for example, organisational issues that could hinder coaching, and dual relationships, for example, recognising the impact and consequences of shared knowledge.

Before discussing these topics in more detail below, the importance of establishing expectations from coaching supervision as a whole and exploring the best hopes from the specific coaching supervision session in question are outlined. This helps the coaching supervision client clarify what topics to bring to coaching supervision.

Establishing Clear Expectations and Agreements for Coaching Supervision

Whatever the topic is that is being brought to coaching supervision, it is important that an initial discussion prior to the start of coaching supervision begins with establishing clarity around a number of aspects. These include but are not limited to:

- the coaching supervision client's expectations,
- the coaching supervision agreement, as outlined in a verbal or written document,
- that the overall purpose of coaching supervision is understood and
- what is and what is not included in the coaching supervision.

This can be done via a co-constructed process so both parties are involved in identifying the specifics of this professional relationship. Any additional items such as confidentiality and the sharing of information with other stakeholders should be addressed within the initial agreement-making stage. This can also serve as an important reminder and anchor, especially when a particular coaching supervision topic is outside the realm of the agreement. Chapter 5 offers more on coaching supervision contracting.

In addition to the ideas mentioned by Clutterbuck et al. (2016) on preparing for coaching supervision, we also recommend that the coaching supervisor creates a form that the coaching supervision client fills out and sends to the coaching supervisor prior to each session to help prepare them for the session. This document could include:

- A reminder of competences

  - The European Mentoring and Coaching Council (EMCC) coaching competences
  - The ICF core competencies for individual coaching
  - The ICF core competencies for team coaching

- Definitions and resources

  - Definitions of coaching supervision
  - Purpose of coaching supervision

- Questions for the coaching supervision client

  - How familiar are you with coaching supervision?
  - Are you bringing any specific case material/a piece from your coaching practice to discuss – is it individual, group or team coaching?
  - Name and brief details of any documents or material you want to explore
  - What are your best hopes from this coaching supervision session?
  - How might the coaching supervisor contribute to you achieving your best hopes?

- What would you like your coaching supervisor to bear in mind/know about you and your coaching?
- Specific focus area in relation to your best hopes:
  - What is already working well?
  - What would you like to improve/develop
  - What questions do you have?
  - What else might you like to say?

Common Topics Arising in Coaching Supervision

The four main functions of coaching supervision have been described previously in Chapter 2. The most common topics brought to coaching supervision are arranged below under each of these areas.

Restorative or Supportive Function

The restorative function in coaching supervision focuses on the well-being of the coaching supervision client to provide care and support in their role as a coach in order to deliver the best coaching experience to their coaching client. This provides a balance between acknowledging the hardship and challenges they face while inviting the coaching supervision client to reflect and integrate their learning in moving forward and connecting with their resources.

Common topics brought by coaching supervision clients in this area include:

- Feeling burdened by their workload
- Reacting negatively to a coaching client and feeling upset
- Exploring a major decision
- Managing a transition
- Uses the sessions as 'crisis management' for their coaching clients
- Processing/exploring emotions related to personal matters, which include

  - Managing anxiety
  - Feeling inadequate or out of their depth
  - Experiencing burnout
  - Struggling with personal issues that impact their work as a coach

Some SF questions and moves that the coaching supervisor can draw on are:

- Asking coping questions:

  - How are you able to manage this situation at this time?
  - What is working, even just a little bit?

- Using the scaling tool – Where are things already? How would you notice signs that things are improving?
- Using metaphors – scaling a mountain, crossing a bridge.

- Instances when the behaviour they want to adopt has occurred already. Gathering rich details around that.
- Using the SF 'moves' and 'gallery' described in Chapter 4 to explore the coaching supervision client's best hopes, preferred future, resourceful past and next steps in relation to the topic.

Professional and Personal Growth

This function of coaching supervision refers to the areas of professional growth that the coaching supervision client identifies that are connected to their skills development, as well as their personal growth related to their values, aspirations and work-life balance.

Common topics here are:

- Improving their confidence as a coach
- Asking for advice in handling tricky situations
- Feeling stuck with a coaching client
- Exploring how to improve work with a certain coaching client
- Honing their professional skills
- Challenges in establishing rapport
- Dealing with a coaching client's lack of progress
- Skills in improving coaching client engagement
- Navigating cultural challenges
- Handling a coaching client's strong emotions
- Feedback on coaching techniques
- Exploring/expanding different coaching approaches
- Working with coaching clients' negative limiting beliefs
- The coaching supervision client launching into psychoanalysing, pathologising and diagnostic language about their coaching client, rather than focusing on exploring their own growth

Some SF questions and moves that the coaching supervisor can draw on are:

- Using SF moves and the gallery (see Chapter 4):

From the ticket office:

- How would you like to explore this so it is helpful for you?
- Suppose we explore this, what difference will it make to you?
- What would you like to take away from our conversation in relation to this?

From the preferred future gallery:

- How would you notice moving forwards with this coaching client?
- How would you notice an improvement in your ability to engage with this coaching client's emotions or navigate the cultural challenges raised?

- What might you be noticing as your skills improve in this area?
- What might your coaching clients be noticing?

From the successful past gallery

- What do you already know about dealing with a similar situation?
- When have things already gone well with this coaching client? What did you notice? How did you do that?

From the giftshop:

- Scale: Where are you now? What would one point higher look like? What would be the first small step towards that?
- What are you taking with you that has been of value to you?
- Discussing and planning an action to make progress

- A general question from Chapter 7 which looks at coaching supervision clients who use different coaching models:

  - What, if any, resources would you like us both to refer to when reflecting on the models/approaches you draw on in your work?

Ethics/Quality Assurance

For this function of coaching supervision, coaching supervisors help to support, guide and promote excellence in the coaching supervision client's ability upholding the professional standards of ethical integrity, excellence and effectiveness, and to promote quality assurance. This benefits the coaching supervision client, their coaching client and the coaching profession as a whole.

Common topics here are:

- Biases towards coaching clients who are different from the coach
- Sharing a mistake or concern regarding ethical considerations
- Making a judgement that impacts the relationship
- Uncertainty about scope of practice/remit and roles between coaching and other modalities
- Managing dual relationships
- Managing contracting and clarity on the coaching agreement
- Confidentiality
- Dealing with self-harm and knowing when to refer to another service
- Unintentionally breaking confidence and sharing information with a third party
- Working with mandated clients and enforcing external goals.

Some SF questions and moves that the coaching supervisor can draw on are: Using the SF 'moves' and 'the gallery'

- What do you already know about this situation and how you might deal with it?

- What have you done already that has helped, even just a little bit?
- What are you certain about already and what would be helpful to address?
- What resources do you have that can help you clarify this? What else do you need?
- On a scale of 1–10, where would you rate your understanding on this already?
- To have all the confidence you need in this situation, what would be helpful to address?
- Would it be alright if I shared my thoughts on this?
- Reviewing ICF and EMCC competencies and codes of ethics and exploring what difference this knowledge makes to handling the situation.

Sometimes the coaching supervisor may be able to take a more indirect approach and explore the coaching supervision client's best hopes in relation to the situation, next steps and so on as normal. However as outlined in Chapter 5 on ethics, sometimes the coaching supervisor may need to step in and be direct, using Thomas' (2011) 'two by four' metaphor, drawing attention to a breach or potential breach in ethics if this has not been noticed by the coaching supervision client. In this case there would need to be a discussion and action plan to address the mistake and rectify the situation to build the relationship between the two parties (Passmore, 2009).

Managerial and Commercial

As outlined in Chapter 2, the managerial and commercial functions of coaching supervision are rarely mentioned. However, the coaching supervision client often experiences concerns and challenges related to business development that can impact their well-being and performance as a coach. It is important therefore that the supervisor explores the business aspect with the coaching supervision client should these arise, providing other functions are also addressed as the main focus for supervision.

Common topics here are:

- Discussing the development of a coaching practice
- Advice on how to expand the coaching client base
- What area of coaching to specialise in
- Working solo or joining a coaching practice
- Pointers and tips on marketing the business
- Market research on what to charge
- Setting up a website, social media and marketing advice

Some strategies that the SF coaching supervisor might offer are:

- Getting a clear idea of what the coaching supervision client wants from the session as a result of the discussion and what makes the topic important.

- I've noticed that you keep circling back to this topic? What is important to you about this? What difference would it make to you and your coaching clients?
- This topic may actually be linked to one of the other functions of coaching supervision such as, not feeling confident which affects their ability, e.g. to write social media posts. Therefore, the same initial topic may lead to exploring improving confidence with one coaching supervision client and with another to giving information about marketing strategies.
- Using the coaching supervision gallery (see Chapter 4) to explore what success would look like in the area of business development (preferred future) and exploring what they already know (successful past) about marketing strategies, knowledge about market trends and practices and so on, and ideas for next steps which may include where they could go to get further information (e.g. a marketing expert).
- The coaching supervisor can share specific information while maintaining the coaching supervision client's autonomy and accountability for implementation. For example, 'These are some of my ideas, what was useful to you from what you heard? How would you like to take this forward?' Suppose you found a way to focus on business development and at the same time focus on the development of your skills as a coach – what difference would this make? Since we've explored this quite a lot, what other topic is of interest to you now?

Transcript with a Supervision Client Wanting to Discuss Business Development

Coaching supervision client:	What I really need to do is to figure out how to start my own coaching business or join one that two of my course mates started, which is going quite well. And then figure out how to build a website and what to charge. Figure out if I want to stick to online coaching because then I can coach anybody. Or stick to direct coaching in person. I need to figure out what to charge too. And another thing is that I'm not sure what area of coaching to focus on. It's making me feel sort of disorganised and all over the place. I'm feeling quite rattled and unsettled. In fact, its making me feel sort of overwhelmed. I'm not sure where to start actually. I want to make some progress on this. Make some decisions.
Coaching supervisor:	There's quite a lot of things you've mentioned here around starting a coaching business. Suppose you get what you need today and start making some progress on this and make some

	decisions. What differences would you start to notice?
Coaching supervision client:	I'd feel like my confident, decisive self. Relief that I had decided some things.
Coaching Supervisor:	Ah ... so when was a recent time you found yourself in a similar situation and somehow, your 'confident, decisive self' stepped in. (Supervisor could also use the scaling tool to explore this.)
Coaching supervision client:	Oh! Well, the last time was when I was looking at all the options about making a new career shift and that's when I decided to take coach training and become a coach.
Coaching supervisor:	How did you do that – decide those things?
Coaching supervision client:	I spent time reviewing the market trends, took some career assessments, saw a career coach and figured out that coaching was what I wanted to do.
Coaching supervisor:	That sounds like a lot of steps you took. What are some ideas that you can take from that experience that might be helpful now?

The coaching supervision client laid out a detailed, step-by-step process that took several months. The coaching supervisor asked questions about the decision-making process and how the coaching supervision client navigated the multi-step process. From this experience, the coaching supervision client eventually figured out a progression of steps and decision points that helped in their current situation. The coaching supervisor also made suggestions regarding additional resources for some of the areas the coaching supervision client was not aware of. Over the course of a few months, the coaching supervision client had made significant progress in the business development of his coaching practice.

Transcript With a Supervision Client Who Arrives With No Topic

Sometimes coaching supervision clients come to coaching supervision with no topic in mind. The pre-session form mentioned earlier in this chapter can provide a gentle nudge to invite the coaching supervision client to reflect and consider how the coaching supervision session can be useful for them. If the questions provided in the form do not spark an idea, the coaching supervisor can use other questions or suggestions about possible options. This transcript addresses several topics raised above and suggested questions and processes in managing them.

Coaching supervisor:	Great to see you! Thanks for coming for coaching supervision today. Know it's a busy period with the holidays. What would you like to focus on today that will be most useful?

Coaching supervision client:	To be honest, even though I read through the pre-session preparation form, I still could not come up with a topic.
Coaching supervisor:	Sure, that happens sometimes. Would it be useful if I ask some questions to see if that sparks anything?
Coaching supervision client:	Yes, that would be helpful.
Coaching supervisor:	We could explore a number of things. We could explore something that has happened recently that impacts where you are today. We could take some time to reflect on that. Or, I could mention a few topics that others have raised. Or we could brainstorm ones that come to mind. What do you think?
Coaching supervision client:	Thanks for that. Actually, what I'm thinking is going on is that one of my clients has been really difficult and it has affected me. I'm not feeling very good about my coaching. In fact, I'm wondering if I should just refer them to someone else.
Coaching supervisor:	I see. So, would that be something you want to talk about today?
Coaching supervision client:	Yes. I wasn't sure if I should bring it up because I'm still sort of hurt by that. But I think that would be really helpful.
Coaching supervisor:	Thank you for being so open and honest about where you are today. As we've worked together for some time, I know you to be a reflective person. It seems to me that you've already been thinking and reflecting on this. How would you like us to explore this?
Coaching supervision client:	I think I want to talk about why I'm so hurt by what happened and why it's affected me so much.
Coaching supervisor:	Ok, sure. And after we explore this a bit today, how are you hoping it would be helpful for you as a coach?
Coaching supervision client:	Well, first I'm really upset with my client and I think they are 'passive-aggressive' and said some things that I think were directed at me but he didn't say it directly about me but sort of insinuated it. I'm trying not to react but I want to talk about the client and how I deal with someone who is 'passive-aggressive'.

Coaching supervisor:	So in discussing this case, how are you hoping it will be helpful for you? What difference do you think it will make for you?
Coaching supervision client:	Well, if I understand the client's behaviour, then I guess I'll know how to deal with their comments to me so I don't react or get flooded.
Coaching supervisor:	What you're saying is that you want to be able to manage your reaction and not get flooded. How would you like to respond instead?
Coaching supervision client:	I guess I wouldn't be trying to analyse him. I'd be calm and composed.
Coaching supervisor:	Suppose, a kind of miracle happened and you respond to him in the way your 'best calm and composed self' would show up. How would you be responding to him differently? What would your client notice?

The session then continued with the coaching supervision client describing the response and behaviour he wanted to embody with some reflections on why his coaching client 'pushed his buttons'. This led to subsequent realisations about the need for managing and containing his reactions to what his coaching client says. The coaching supervision client experienced a shift in perception of his coaching client and away from analysing and diagnosing the situation. The coaching supervision client's demeanour changed from 'beating himself up' to one of 'composure and confidence', which were descriptions of what he wanted.

Many of these questions from the transcript have elements of useful skills and tools the coaching supervisor can apply across the board to most if not all common topics raised in this chapter. While the exact questions are tailored to a specific topic, the use of the question or 'moves' and 'the gallery' can be applied in any coaching supervision conversation.

Asking for Advice

This topic is one that surfaces for the coaching supervision clients across all the different coaching supervision functions. While the usual response of an SF coaching supervisor is 'to pull the wisdom from the therapist [coach] rather than tell them what to do' (Pichot & Dolan, 2003, p. 173), 'effective supervisors must acquire the ability to determine when they need to provide information' (Pichot & Dolan, 2003, p. 171).

A transcript of a coaching supervision session is shown below, where the coaching supervision client is stuck and asking for advice. How an SF coaching supervisor offers advice when needed was also shown in the transcript of case coaching supervision in Chapter 6. Here another approach is shown, where the coaching supervision client is asked what difference being given the right advice would make. This is useful to help the coaching supervision client to deal with the case they are bringing and also offers parallel learning that can occur for the coaching supervision client as they also face a similar situation in which their coaching client is seeking advice.

Coaching supervision client:	So, I'm sort of stuck because the client is asking me for advice on what she should do. And whichever way she goes does not bring much relief. And I'm afraid to tell her what to do because I know that is not part of coaching. I guess what I want is some advice from you on how to handle this tricky situation.
Coaching supervisor:	Yes, I can see why this would be challenging for you, given the situation you've described. There's a lot of moving pieces here, as you said.
Coaching supervision client:	Yes! And if I give her the wrong advice, what will happen then? And if I don't help her, that's not good either.
Coaching supervisor:	So, we've explored some of the things you've done already in helping her navigate this situation. I'm wondering how confident you are that you've explored everything to your satisfaction?
Coaching supervision client:	The only thing left that I can come up with is just telling her what to do. Because we've been working on this for months now and nothing has shifted for her.
Coaching supervisor:	Yes, I see you've told me about six different things you've explored with her.
Coaching supervision client:	Yes, I'm really stuck.
Coaching supervisor:	I'm wondering, suppose I offer you the best advice ever, what difference do you suppose it would make for you?
Coaching supervision client:	Well, I would feel like I've done all I can to help her.
Coaching supervisor:	What else?
Coaching supervision client:	I guess I do feel a lot of sympathy towards her and don't want her to suffer. She has endured a lot through this situation. She is quite a spitfire girl. She has a high capacity for enduring the 'shit' and keeps showing up for work. Her boss is a nightmare, I tell you. I wouldn't say that to her, but he really is.
Coaching supervisor:	What's important to you, then, is that you know you've done all you can to help her. How come this is important to you?

Coaching supervision client:	Good question ... I'm starting to think that maybe I'm getting too emotionally caught up in this. Hmmm ...
Coaching supervisor:	What's coming to your mind as you say that?
Coaching supervision client:	Yeah, well ... I'm trying so hard to help her and maybe I need to step back a bit.
Coaching supervisor:	And how would 'stepping back' be helpful for you?
Coaching supervision client:	I think I need to take a more objective view – maybe I'm getting lost in the forest for the trees. Maybe I'm trying to solve her problem. Hmmmm.
Coaching supervisor:	Where are you now in this exploration of offering advice?
Coaching supervision client:	Seems to me that she wants advice to help her resolve her situation and now I'm asking you for advice because I want to resolve this. Very interesting!
Coaching supervisor:	Well, what do you think will be a good way forward for you?
Coaching supervision client:	I need to think about this 'being stuck'. I've forgotten my role as a coach, I think. I remember in my coaching course some time ago, 'not to take my client's monkeys'. And I think I sort of did.
Coaching supervisor:	Oh, I love that. 'Don't take your client's monkeys'. So, instead of taking their monkeys, what do you want to do? How do you want to manage this?
Coaching supervision client:	I think I need to step back, take her monkey off my back and not get caught up in her web.
Coaching supervisor:	And in doing that, what is your idea of how you want to move forward today?
Coaching supervision client:	I think I was feeling insecure because I didn't know how to give her advice on her tricky situation.
Coaching supervisor:	And what are you more sure about now?
Coaching supervision client:	I think I need to go back to the coaching agreement. Re-establish what she wants from our coaching session. Because if she had said 'I want advice' on this, I would not have taken that on. I know that now.
Coaching supervisor:	What else has surfaced for you in how to manage this situation that you feel confident about?

The coaching supervision client continues to discuss the need to take a step back and stay out of the coaching client's web of confusion. This led to reflections about his role and needing to partner with her to clarify the desired outcomes from their coaching. This reminded him what the original coaching goal had been. And likewise, with the coaching supervisor, the discussion was around how the coaching supervision client would manage to 'stay out of the web' and surface the coaching client's ability to manage and cope with an on-going work situation. The coaching supervision client later reported that his coaching client had discovered her tolerance to the 'shit' was a way of coping and realised there were more good reasons to stay where she was versus trying to solve something that had no resolution that was within her control, except that of her ability for resilience.

Common Topics in Team Coaching Supervision

Chapter 13 covers team coaching supervision in detail and states that team coaching supervision addresses the co-creation of the relationship with the team of the coaching supervision client related to the team coaching experience. The similarities between coaching supervision focused on team and individual coaching are that the focus of the coaching supervision is on the coaching supervision client and not on the coaching client. The differences are in the topics and needs of the coaching supervision client to enhance the work they do.

Common topics brought to team coaching supervision include:

- contracting – contracting with the sponsor that differs from contracting with the team,
- contracting team coaching services when the team is in need of something else,
- contracting when the buyer of team coaching doesn't have a clear understanding of team coaching,
- reflecting on the team coach's ongoing learning,
- challenges faced in the team coaching process and
- responding to the evolving needs of the teams they work with.

These three areas of common topics in team coaching supervision are discussed under the same categories as are used in Chapter 13:

- the co-creation of relationships – with the team or teams that the team coach is engaging with,
- the process – either the overall team coaching process or the process within a team coaching workshop and
- the knowledge – be it specific team coaching knowledge or allied knowledge such as facilitation skills.

Some strategies that the SF coaching supervisor might offer are:

As detailed earlier in this chapter, the SF gallery is an effective frame for exploring issues related to personal and professional growth that are brought by coaching supervision clients. The SF gallery can also be used to explore issues that are brought to coaching supervision by team coaching supervision clients. The following are some variations of questions that can be used in such contexts:

- Ticket office
  - Let's explore together the specific areas you would like to focus on during our team coaching supervision. What aspects of your professional identity and practice are you keen to develop?
  - What part of your work would you like to reflect on today? And what would you like to be different going forwards in relation to this?

- Preferred future
  - As you imagine yourself at your best in your team coaching practice, what would that look like in terms of your relationship with the team members? What would the team notice with you at your best? What would be different in how you interact with the team? What would be different in what you feel, think and do?

- Successful/past resources (drawing on past experiences as individual or team coaches)
  - When have you had a similar experience with an individual coaching client? What was useful back then?
  - When was a past experience where you faced a similar challenge to what you are encountering now in your team coaching practice? How did you manage that situation successfully and how might you apply those lessons learned in your current context?

  Gift shop:

  'What have you learned so far from your reflections on this team and your interactions with them?'

  'What might you want to do to further prepare yourself for the next time you engage with this team?'

Reflection Exercise

- What are the most common topics and challenges that you face as a coaching supervisor?
- Please choose two topics from the lists above or choose one of your own.

  - What would be some SF questions and moves to support the learning and growth of the coaching supervision client in this situation?

References

Clutterbuck, D., Whitaker, C., & Lucas, M. (2016). *Coaching supervision: A practical guide for supervisees*. Routledge.

Hawkins, P., Turner, E., & Passmore, J. (2019). *The manifesto for supervision*. Henley Business School and Association for Coaching.

McAnally, K., Abrams, L., Asmus, M. J., & Hildebrandt, T. (2020). *Global coaching supervision. A study of the perceptions and practices around the world*. International Coaching Federation. Retrieved from https://researchportal.coachingfederation.org/Document/Pdf/abstract_3516

Passmore, J. (2009). Coaching ethics: Making ethical decisions: Experts and novices. *The Coaching Psychologist. 5*(1), 2.

Passmore, J., & McGoldrick, S. (2009). Super-vision, extra-vision or blind faith? A grounded theory study of the efficacy of coaching supervision. *International Coaching Psychology Review. 4*(2), 145–161.

Pichot, T., & Dolan, Y. M. (2003). *Solution-focused brief therapy: Its effective use in agency settings*. The Haworth Press Inc.

Thomas, F. N. (2011). Semaphore, metaphor, … two-by-four. In T.S. Nelson (Ed). *Doing something different. Solution-focused brief therapy practices* (pp. 243–248). Routledge.

15 Suppose a Miracle Happened

Our Preferred Future for Coaching Supervision

Kirsten Dierolf and Svea van der Hoorn

Introduction

"Suppose a miracle happened ... what might then become possible?" is one of the traditional ways practitioners of Solution Focused (SF) coaching invite a description of the preferred future. In this chapter, we revisit the chapters of this book on Solution Focused coaching supervision and provide our vision, our preferred future for each. Since SF coaching supervision is an emerging field, there is much that can be developed and researched. We sincerely hope that the field will grow both in theory and in practice. Our hopes are expressed in this chapter.

Our Best Hopes for the Future of Coaching Supervision

Coaching supervision is an emergent field. We invite coaches and coaching supervisors to co-construct customised conversations that help each coach participating in coaching supervision to learn and grow. As we mentioned at the beginning of this book, coaching supervision is a family resemblance concept. The conversations that are being conducted under the heading of coaching supervision are very diverse. Coaching supervisors and coaching supervision clients come from different models and theories of change, and different socio-economic and political worlds. Coaches entering coaching supervision have different levels of maturity in their practice and serve a wide diversity of clients. Coaching supervision fulfils many different functions. It is therefore necessary and desirable to keep the field of coaching supervision diverse, complex and welcoming of difference. It is desirable that we make space for as many forms of coaching supervision as may be helpful to coaching supervision clients. And we need to do this without becoming fragmented, without having no or only a vague identity and without excusing the field for being a philosophical and methodological mess and muddle.

Accreditation agencies like European Mentoring and Coaching Council (EMCC) and International Coaching Federation (ICF) are endeavouring to work towards quality assurance of coaching supervision and the professionalisation of the field. We sincerely hope that this process of professionalisation of coaching supervision will find ways to acknowledge and appreciate the diversity of coaching supervision. If you asked us whether we want only

DOI: 10.4324/9781003390527-15

SF coaching supervisors on the planet you would hear a resounding "No!". We want every coaching supervision client to find the coaching supervisor that they can trust, and who can help them develop in the way that they would like to develop. While we appreciate thinking that is in favour of coaching supervision core competencies, we hope that these frameworks can be revisited and refined to expand the awareness of philosophical coherence. This would reduce the current bias against social constructionist approaches, which we view as probably due to lack of awareness or a lack of critical thinking about the philosophical homes of the various coaching and coaching supervision models. A tomato may be classifiable as a fruit, but few would welcome it being added to a fruit salad. We would hope that more awareness about the different philosophies underpinning coaching supervision and coaching can become part of mainstream discussion and debate and that individualised and essentialist psychologies can stop being regarded as the unquestionable panacea for all things coaching and coaching supervision.

Coaches who wish to gain a credential from the ICF have to submit one or two recordings in which they demonstrate their capability to coach in ways that allow assessors to detect the ICF core competencies. Whether this process is really a good assessment of applicants' competence or a reliable sample of their daily coaching is debatable. Coaching supervision is even more customised and diverse. We really hope that the ICF will not choose a similar path towards the credentialing of coaching supervisors, as has been followed to date in the creation and revision of the core competency model. Job analysis is not questioned as a methodology (Voskuijl, 2017). Rather its suitability as a method for analysis of an activity characterised by the co-creation of shared meanings and understandings by those involved in the conversation is questioned. We are encouraged at the importance given to partnering in the ICF definition of coaching and in the criteria for assessment of coaching competencies, namely the behaviourally anchored ratings scales (BARS) for the Associate Certified Coach (ACC) and Master Certified Coach (MCC) credentials, and the markers for the Professional Certified Coach (PCC).

Theory and Research

We would like to see a rigorous review of communication theory and hope for a move to going beyond the sender-receiver and even the sender-blackbox-receiver model. We would welcome consideration of Wittengenstein's concept of language games, namely, that communication involves concrete social activities that crucially involve the use of specific forms of language (Peters, 2020). Similarly, we are of the view that much can be learned about partnering in coaching from the microanalysis research, in particular around the idea of listening being able to be non-directive (Bavelas & Gerwing, 2011).

> Research showed that addressees who were not distracted used a wide variety of behaviors to contribute to dialogue without interrupting the

speaker, such as brief vocalizations, facial displays, and even gestures. Speakers and addressees regulated the timing of addressee responses using an interactive pattern of gaze. Addressees also indicated understanding by their formulations, which summarized or paraphrased what the speaker had said. However, our analysis showed that these formulations were not neutral. The analysis of addressees in face-to-face dialogue generates a deeper understanding of the listening process and has implications for listening in applied settings, such as psychotherapy or health care interactions.

(Bavelas & Gerwing, 2011, p. 179)

We would welcome such a shift in how communication, and in particular partnering between speakers engaged in a coaching conversation, is viewed. We see such a shift as timeous and possibly even evolutionary for coaching and coaching supervision. It would bring to a pause the over dominance of psychological theory in the development of what are considered to be detectable signs of good coaching. A repository of microanalysis research publications can be found on Janet Bavelas' website (Bavelas, n.d.).

Our preferred future includes increasing the qualitative research studies conducted into the experience of coaching supervisors and their coaching supervision clients. Also, we see that there is a great need to find out what is actually going on coaching supervision, rather than to rely on accounts of what happens in coaching supervision. There is a lot of space for thorough analysis of co-construction as it takes place in coaching supervision. Janet Bavelas' work on the microanalysis of face-to-face dialogue (e.g. Bavelas et al., 2000, 2014, 2017) provides a start. In the light of this research, what needs a major re-think by accreditation agencies is the insistence on the use of audio only recordings when assessing coaching capability. This applies equally to coaching supervision where coaching supervisors and their coaching supervision clients refer to transcripts and/or audio recordings of coaching that was undertaken in a face-to-face setting. Face-to-face dialogue review has made clear the significance of co-speech gestures, such as facial expressions and hand gestures, in the co-construction of the conversation.

Apart from research into practice we would love to see more clarity with regard to the different strands of coaching supervision. We would like to see more historical work and also more work differentiating the different theoretical approaches. We would support a growing awareness and multilogue around how our theories and assumptions shape the work that we are doing. We believe that we always speak from our own perspective, including our theoretical orientation, and that only when we become aware of these theoretical assumptions can we talk meaningfully with other practitioners and theorists who hold different assumptions. We sincerely hope that these exchanges between practitioners from different approaches will result in the development of the coaching profession in general and coaching supervision in particular.

Individual Solution Focused Coaching Supervision

More research and practice of coaching supervision which includes stakeholders from the coaching supervision client's environment are needed. If we are assuming that a coaching supervisor not only supports an individual coaching supervision client to grow, but is also there to promote the thriving of the whole coaching relationship, then doing more supervision in collaboration with the complexity of the client's environment is called for.

Solution Focused, Narrative, Interactional and other collaborative practitioners of the helping professions have just started talking to one another. We want to see these relationships grow and we would like the field to harvest the fruits of the interactions of social constructionist and other practitioners as they engage in critical debates about their practices, their thinking and their good reasons for adopting the theories and the models that they draw on.

Demonstrating Ethical Coaching Practice

In short, we want to see more engagement with ethics – in coach education, in coaching supervision, in everyday coaching. We support coaches and coaching supervisors regarding engagement with ethics as necessary for self-regulation and accountability in one's practice, and not as a compliance with external regulation.

Coupled to this is the question of at what time intervals and in response to what prompts and trends do coaching accreditation agencies review their definitions of coaching, their Codes of Ethics, their statements about diversity, equity and inclusion, and about current issues, such as climate change? The criteria against which coaching and coaching supervision are quality assured have mostly been about asking those engaged in these activities to formulate the standards. We would welcome a move to gather data from buyers and recipients of services, for example, as has been done in research into patients' experience and recommendations for hospitals and community service centres (National Institute for Health and Care Research, 2020).

This would then add to and be integrated into the data sets from which coaching and coaching supervision accreditation agencies develop standards of practice and assessment criteria. Deliberate Practice (see Chapter 8) has much to offer as a way to gather relevant and appropriate client data.

Finally, there is an urgent need to re-consider the scope and remit pertaining to coaching. Those coaches and coaching supervisors who are duty bound to uphold a Code of Ethics are also bound by scope and remit restrictions. Some are explicit, and some implied. The COVID-19 crisis of the early 2020s provided lived experience of what coaches may face as what coaching clients expect from them when the clients' worlds are already significantly disrupted. Many coaches and coaching supervisors faced ethical dilemmas to which the recommended referral to other services was not a solution. Other services were disrupted from operating, inaccessible due to travel restrictions and physical distancing requirements, but most importantly, clients did not wish to be sent outside of a relationship characterised by the cultivation of mutual trust and respect, and hence safety. It beholds the coaching profession as a whole, and the coaching and coaching supervision accreditation agencies to draw on this period in our history to create updated guidelines on the scope and remit for coaches, including how to fulfil ethical coaching requirements when referral to alternate services is not an immediately viable option.

Case Supervision

We would like to see it become the norm in case supervision that there is less talking about the client and more talking about the coaching supervision client in relation to who needs to be or do differently when the coaching is stuck. This is not because of a shift in blame but in response to a shift in responsibility, which has ethical implications. The coaching supervisor who holds a focus on "what are your best hopes about how you would like to see yourself serving this coaching client well?" invites a significantly different focus on attention for the coaching supervision. This is followed by enquiries around what the coaching supervision client is already doing that the coaching client is responding to with learning and growth. Then the coaching supervision conversation may shift even more to the interactional focus with questions about the coaching supervision client's contributions to the coaching conversation, and how they can be or do something different that is likely to shift the engagement towards their best hopes.

In particular, we would welcome a re-think and expansion around the concept of reluctance and resistance. The dominance of psychological theory that privileges intrapsychic explanations has resulted in reluctance and resistance often being located as if inside the client (coaching client and coaching supervision client). We would welcome a more interactional view where reluctance and resistance are considered as a "between" phenomenon, and hence the coaching supervision client and the coaching supervisor looking to their contributions to reluctance and resistance. We would also support a view that reluctance and resistance are usual experiences in human relationships, and not automatically signs of deficit, dysfunction or pathology. We invite a visit or for some readers, a re-visit of the by now regarded as old, but for the SF approach considered seminal, namely the 1984 paper "Death of Resistance" (de Shazer, 1984). For those keen to stay with a psychological approach to coaching supervision, and looking for something beyond the cognitivist psychology focus that has been prevalent, we invite exploration of discursive psychology, with its focus on communication as a social activity (Martínez-Guzmána et al., 2016; Wiggins, 2017).

Supervision of Other Clients With Other Coaching Models

Given some of our best hopes expressed above, we welcome the continuation of a variety of coaching supervision approaches, models and practices. What we do not support is that some are privileged as being necessarily better than others. This is an unfortunate but intentional consequence of the best practice proposition. We support that coaching supervisors should inform their practice with findings from outcomes and effectiveness research, but not at the cost of de-contextualising or marginalising forms of coaching supervision that may not be within the dominant or mainstream paradigm. We welcome innovation that is philosophically explicit and coherent, that draws on methodologically sound and coherent research, that is context aware and responsive, and that serves the coaching supervisor and coaching supervision client in offering a quality coaching experience to the wide variety of clients that coaches engage with.

From an SF perspective we remain appreciative of taking a not-knowing stance in coaching supervision in relation to the expertise that coaching supervision clients bring to their coaching supervision conversations. Our appreciation of their expertise, and our commitment to partnering and equity, does not equal knowing nothing. However, we offer our expertise as a resource from which we can draw in the coaching supervision, together with the accountability to share with our coaching supervision clients an evidence trail that makes accessible how we know what we know.

We will continue to regard coaching supervision as serving the coaching supervision client well when the coaching supervisor holds a focus on the coaching supervision client becoming more competent and hence confident in knowing their own model, and developing learning and growth plans to become even better at their own coaching approach/model. If a coaching supervision client wishes to expand their expertise, we would welcome coaching supervisors actively encouraging further training in particular models/ approaches, rather than the growing tendency to consider an online search, attending a webinar or few as sufficient to claim expertise in a model/approach. We would welcome the coaching education community to offer some guidelines in response to the "how long is a piece of string" question that many coaches and coaching supervisors ask. This question about how much coaching education is sufficient to claim expertise to practice is an ethical question of legitimacy and a reputational question of credibility. It should not be responded to primarily as a commercial or branding question, but rather as a quality assurance, ethical promise to buyers of coaching and coaching clients.

Deliberate Practice and Reflective Practice

Deliberate Practice has been shown to support the development of excellence in many fields. We hope to see more research that generates large data sets of client feedback. This calls for collaborative research efforts between agencies and institutions that have the capacity for large data set research and can ensure appropriate data privacy and protection. We would be dismayed if the trend to use client feedback for performance management of coaches gains even more momentum. The criteria used by agencies including coaching platforms could be significant sources of data if, and only if, they are premised on the actuality that coaching conversations are co-constructed and hence require a nuanced and theoretically coherent approach to the generation of the data gathering tools, the data processing and analysis methods, and the claims made about findings. We hope to see an increase in the use of measures such as the Session Rating Scale (Miller et al., 2002) and the Outcome Rating Scale (Miller & Duncan, 2000).

We would be delighted to see Deliberate Practice becoming as established as is its natural companion Reflective Practice. An expansion in Reflective Practice that we would welcome is to go beyond the coaching supervision tendency to focus reflection on the coaching supervision client's inner emotions to include an equal focus on interactional reflection on what is happening between the people involved in the coaching. This includes but is not limited to clients, buyers of coaching and stakeholders who stand to benefit or be disadvantaged by the outcomes of the coaching.

To make it more likely that coaching supervisors and coaching supervision clients would make use of Reflective and Deliberate Practice, we would like to see more structures/guidelines like those provided and illustrated in Chapter 9 on Reflective Practice.

Mentor Coaching

As mentioned earlier, we would welcome the re-consideration of the value and appropriateness of video, audio, transcript analysis and reflection logs in the ICF mentor coaching process, as well as in coaching supervision in general. This is an appropriate collaborative project for the coaching accreditation agencies, as well as for academic and research institutions involved in coaching education and development, as well as in communications research. This would help to take coaching from being regarded as a question and answer language game, to a social activity aimed at development via learning and growth.

Given that ICF mentor coaching forms part of the assessment protocol used to admit or refuse coaches access to ICF credentials, the ICF is well placed to also look into ethical guidelines for data protection and security, in particular in relation to artificial intelligence (AI) tools that many mentor coaches are already utilising to reduce the labour intensity of the mentor coaching activity. This includes the use of AI tools for analysing transcripts to detect the presence of ICF core competencies. Investigation of the extent to which such tools further entrench the idea that coaching is a question and answer language game would be welcomed as a service to coaching supervisor whose focus is more on getting on with their practice than researching emerging trends.

Group Supervision and Peer Supervision

We welcome an increase in the use of group and peer coaching supervision as a way to take collective accountability of the diversity, equity, inclusion, belonging and social justice agenda. With the rise of online access and easy-to-use low-cost language translation tools, coaching supervision clients have significantly increased access to colleagues and coaching supervisors. The segmentation that time zones create continues to encourage silos and coaching supervisors are encouraged to set themselves the challenge of being willing to engage at least a few times a year in webinars and professional coaching activities that take them to worlds that are beyond their everyday experience.

As the market becomes increasingly flooded with coaches, there may well be implications for the range of income generation for coaches. We welcome an awareness and respect for that coaching exists not only in the commercially driven corporate world but also in the worlds of communities and individual lives. Group and peer supervision allow coaches more equitable-for-all access to coaching supervision. Coaching supervisors have generally invested considerable time and money in their own education and expertise development. Being able to continue to earn their desired income while enabling coaching supervision clients to share the cost burden is for us an ethical trend we would like to see flourish.

Team Coaching Supervision

Team coaching has been alive and well for decades, despite it becoming the latest shiny bright object in the early 2020s. Whenever something becomes a trend it attracts attention and creates commercial opportunity. We would like to see that those well versed in individual coaching and coaching supervision for those who work with an individual client in coaching sessions exercise restraint from assuming that their expertise is automatically transferable to coaching supervision for those who are coaching teams. Yes there is transferability, and, no, we do not regard experience in only individual coaching and individual coaching supervision as sufficient to offer team coaching supervision. Paradoxically, we do not regard it as necessary that the coaching supervisor have team coaching experience. This would go against the principles of what we described in Chapter 7 on offering coaching supervision to coaching supervision clients that coach in a model/approach different from what is familiar to the supervisor.

The main shift we would like to see is the rise in awareness of engagement with the interactional communication and behavioural web that is part of every team's everyday operational life. We propose that there is complexity, uncertainty and ambiguity that can be well responded to by adapting an interactional approach. We note the rising trend to make use of AI by team coaches as a way to manage the complexity, uncertainty and ambiguity. Advancements in emerging technologies and the way Large Language Models and Artificial Intelligence (AI) can be embedded in team coaching are an example. This raises ethical questions about whether what makes things easier is necessarily offering an ethical coaching service? A spin off is that coaching supervisors may well face increasing requests to discuss the ethics of using AI in team coaching and may well feel out of their depth at the level of knowledge to support their team coaching supervision clients to make informed ethical decisions. This will confront coaching supervisors with expanding their resource and knowledge networks or to accept that when one tries to be all things to all people, one often risks becoming nothing to no one. We would welcome a move towards explicit communication by those offering team coaching supervision about what is within the scope and remit of what they offer, particularly when it comes to the gatekeeper and guru functions of coaching supervision as outlined by Thomas (2013).

We would welcome more research into coaching supervision specifically focused on being of service to team coaches.

What and How Now?

Our intention in writing this book was to contribute to and create value for a diversity of readers, including but not limited to aspirant coaches, those already coaching, coaching supervisors, coaching supervision clients, academics, researchers, subject matter experts, coach education providers and anyone who is drawn to the idea that through purposeful conversations, we can create a world of words within which people can learn and grow.

For those who would like to explore a deeper dive into the SF approach, we invite you to visit the Solutions Academy playlists available on YouTube. The one playlist offers descriptions and illustrations of the SF principles and work in action (SolutionsAcademy, 2021). The other offers an exploration of the ICF core competencies (SolutionsAcademy, 2023).

We hope that you have been inspired, perhaps disturbed, by your reading journey with this book. We would be glad if it leads to activity on your part that invigorates you, your work and is of service to those you engage with.

References

Bavelas, J. B. (n.d.). *Janet Beavin Bavelas Publications.* Retrieved February 26, 2024, from http://web.uvic.ca/psyc/bavelas

Bavelas, J. B., Coates, L., & Johnson, T. (2000). Listeners as co-narrators. *Journal of Personality and Social Psychology 79*(6), 941–952.

Bavelas, J. B., & Gerwing, J. (2011). The listener as addressee in face-to-face dialogue. *International Journal of Listening 25*(3), 178–198.

Bavelas, J. B., De Jong, P., Smock Jordan, S., & Korman, H. (2014). The theoretical and research basis of co-constructing meaning in dialogue. *Journal of Solution-Focused Brief Therapy 2*(2), 1–24.

Bavelas, J. B., Gerwing, J., Healing, S., & Tomori, C. (2017). Microanalysis of face-to-face dialogue (MFD). In D.L. Worthington & G. Bodie (Eds.), *The sourcebook of listening methodology & measurement* (pp. 445–452). John Wiley & Sons.

de Shazer, S. (1984). Death of resistance. *Family Process 23*(1), 11–21.

Martínez-Guzmána, A., Stecherb, A., & Lupicinio Íñiguez-Ruedac, L. (2016). Discursive psychology contributions to qualitative research in social psychology: An analysis of its ethnomethodological heritage. *Psicologia USP 27*(3), 510–520.

Miller, S. D., & Duncan, B. L. (2000). *The Outcome Rating Scale.* Author.

Miller, S. D., Duncan, B. L., & Johnson, L. D. (2002). *The Session Rating Scale 3.0.* Author.

National Institute for Health and Care Research (2020). Improving care by using patient feedback. Retrieved from https://evidence.nihr.ac.uk/collection/improving-care-by-using-patient-feedback/. https://doi.org/10.3310/themedreview-04237

Peters, M. A. (2020). Language-games philosophy: Language-games as rationality and method. *Educational Philosophy and Theory 54*(12), 1929–1935. https://doi.org/10.1080/00131857.2020.1821190

SolutionsAcademy (2021, September 3). *SolutionsAcademy Playlist – Solution Focus: Solution Focused principles and the work in action.* [YouTube Channel]. YouTube. https://www.youtube.com/playlist?list=PLesodpDjOte6gR0id6LwF5SDLIK n6G_1_

SolutionsAcademy (2023, April 4). *SolutionsAcademy Playlist of ICF core competencies explained.* [YouTube Channel]. YouTube. https://www.youtube.com/playlist?list=PLesodpDjOte76Q0L91tmqz53kIljcf340

Thomas, F. N. (2013). *Solution-focused supervision: A resource-oriented approach to developing clinical expertise.* Springer.

Voskuijl, O. F. (2017). Job analysis: Current and future perspectives. In A. Evers, N. Anderson, & O.F. Voskuijl (Eds.), *The Blackwell handbook of personnel selection.* Blackwell. https://doi.org/10.1002/9781405164221.ch2

Wiggins, S. (2017). *Discursive psychology: Theory, method and applications.* SAGE. https://doi.org/10.4135/9781473983335

Appendix
Transcript of Group Supervision Using the Reflecting Team Approach

This transcript is from a recording of a demonstration of the reflecting team process made by the authors for training purposes.

The supervisor starts by reminding the group of the process.

Coaching supervisor: Welcome, everybody. We're going to use a reflecting team format today. Debbie will share a case with us today that she needs some help with. So just a reminder for how we're going to be proceeding. She will start by sharing her case and expressing the help she needs. Then we'll have a round where one by one we will ask clarifying questions. Then a round of appreciation – what did we notice that she did well. And then the final stage, we will reflect and offer something useful for her to take away: an idea, a story, an aphorism, a poem. And then she will respond by sharing what she's taking away from this reflecting team process. So, Debbie, you'll start things off.

Stages 1 and 2: Preparing and Presenting

The aim is for the presenter to first share what their hopes from the supervision are, as this then helps the reflecting team listen for what might be helpful to the coach. However it is common, as here, that the coach launches straight into describing the case. The facilitator may then need to politely interrupt or ask again what the coach wants feedback on before proceeding.

Coaching supervision client (Debbie): This involves a young man, maybe late 20s. We've had a couple of sessions and I'm stuck, going around in circles. This young man comes from a very colourful past. Very good looking, lots of tats, body piercings and wild hair. And he's trying to make a change in his life and work in a business situation. He's got an entrepreneur relationship with lots of different things he's doing. And now he's really focused and he wants to go into a business. So the business school he wanted to sign up for wouldn't allow him because he didn't meet the qualification. But because of the calibre of person he is, he went to talk to the admissions person and made a personal appeal. And they accepted him. So, when he's clear on what he wants, he goes after it, whether it's good or bad. So he, really, wants to take this leadership training. He started the programme. The other aspect is he talks about his relationships like girlfriend, his dad as one in which he's very different from everyone else temperamentally. And he gets personally offended or hurt. And all his relationships telling him, "let it go, you're too sensitive". He was referred by his friend originally. So he's in my office because if he's going to go into business, he knows he needs to address some things about who he is. And he's in turmoil about how come he has trouble letting things go. And he keeps deferring to me with "What would be your advice? How can I let go?" And I catch myself sometimes. "Well, it sounds like letting go is a good idea". And then I catch myself from falling into that trap and trying to really stay in that space. He is this interesting mixture of very mature, clear and driven and almost emotionally needy. So there's this tendency to have a kind of a motherly response to what I consider as emotional affirmation. And I'm stuck because I'm wondering, I've seen him for two sessions. Are we getting anywhere? In terms of the coaching agreement, I thought we were clear, but we seem to be sort of vacillating back and forth. So I'm really stuck and I'm not sure how to proceed.

Coaching supervisor: So, Debbie, just to be clear, what would help you from this session?

Coaching supervision client: I'm stuck on how to proceed. I'm wondering, do I recalibrate the goal? What would be a good way to engage again? I feel like I've lost my way.

Coaching supervisor:	Well, thank you for sharing. Now I would like to invite the team one by one to ask any clarifying questions that would help you understand the case.

Stage 3: Clarifying

Jane:	Could you share Debbie, about what the actual coaching agreement is? What does he want to be different as a result of these sessions?
Coaching supervision client:	His question was, "Is he emotionally weak and vulnerable, which is not a good thing when you're going to enter the business world. What can he do to develop some strength or confidence?" So that idea of confidence.
Chris:	You mentioned that his friend suggested him for coaching, but I'm not sure if he wants to be at the coaching or if this is his friend pushing him into the coaching.
Coaching supervision client:	At the beginning he was maybe exploring would therapy be the right thing. And I think as we rolled along, because we had a discussion around what we can and can't do. If it's going to be therapy, then you need to find someone who can do that. If we do coaching, it's what do you want to grow and develop. So we came to the idea of confidence, which was something he wanted to work on. It was no longer, "My friend thinks I could benefit". So there was a shift.
Kirsten:	Have you thought about doing the Hogan assessment? I think that would be just wonderful.
Coaching supervision client:	Yes, I thought of that.

The supervisor needs to gently intervene here to remind the coaches that at this stage the questions are for clarification here not making suggestions yet.

Coaching supervisor:	Hang in there a minute. At this stage of our process, we're simply trying to seek clarification about the case, not suggesting ideas.
Kirsten:	Okay. Sorry.
Coaching supervisor:	No problem. So please feel free to ask any clarifying question about the nature of the case or what Debbie is trying.

Svea:	I'm wondering about the bigger frame. You say you've had two sessions with him. Have you contracted for a particular number of sessions?
Coaching supervision client:	I asked him that question and he said, let's just take it one session at a time. And so I honestly don't know, within the session, you know, is he going to come back until at the end he'll say, I'll get in touch with you or let's go ahead and schedule one. So I'm realising I have a bit of insecurity. I'm not even sure that's the right way to proceed either. Maybe I need to have an agreement about, let's do four sessions. That's what I need feedback about.
Cristina:	Debbie, you said at some point something about this motherly attitude and his need for all of those feelings. Then you spoke about you don't know if it's supposed to be coaching or therapy. How do you feel that it fits with coaching or with therapy?
Coaching supervision client:	So I try to be very clear about the differences so I don't have any conflict in the way that I'm proceeding. At one point, I gave him an affirmation of what I heard, and he wept. And he said, I've never had anyone compliment me like that. And that kind of opened up this, this hurt where his mum always criticised him. And so then I said, do you feel like this is something you want to explore in therapy or how would you like to carry on? And that was a turning point. So I felt like I'm on the right track because I affirmed what I heard about his good side. Even though he's always labelled as a rebel and criticised for getting into trouble. I said for someone to convince a world class business programme to accept them, there has to be something they saw in you. So I feel like complimenting is very helpful. That builds his confidence. But there is a part of me that's wondering, does he need more support?
Coaching supervisor:	Okay. Any other clarifying questions?
Sukanya:	Debbie, you had said at the beginning something about this young man asking how he can let go of things. Could you clarify what that meant?

Coaching supervision client:	He described to me that in a conversation, maybe his girlfriend or his dad or his friends, and all of a sudden someone says something and then it's like it pricks him. He obsesses and ruminates about it. And because I was worried does he have some psychological problems with that? And as we explored it, what emerged was his desire for perfectionism. This is something that no one has picked up on in his life. They saw him as a loser. So I felt like this was an important aspect that we explored, is the letting go so that he can see if others do criticise or see something that's inadequate. He sees it as an opportunity for growth, and that brought some tears. So getting to know himself and building the confidence around these very deeply seated emotional things. That seemed to help him make progress. But am I exploring things that are in the coaching realm? And so while he seems to be making progress, I need to know I am doing my ethical duty also.
Coaching supervisor:	Any other clarifying questions?
Jane:	Debbie, you say you were struggling with giving advice and knowing that that's not coaching. But can you share how you responded when he said, what do you think I should do?
Coaching supervision client:	The first time I just fell into it and gave him advice. "Sounds like you need to let go". And then I caught myself. Because I get caught up in his emotion and in how tender and vulnerable he is. But there's this other great aspect of who he wants to grow into.

Stage 4: Affirming

Coaching supervisor:	If there are no other clarifying questions, then we'll move into this next phase of expressing what we've appreciated about what we've heard Debbie doing.
Chris:	I really appreciate Debbie bringing so vulnerably and openly this case to us. And also saying, I understand that this is not the way to coach. These are the things that I'd like to do better. And recognising how vulnerable the client could be in this situation, especially dealing with what sounds like some difficulties for him

as he's maturing into a young man and dealing with the real issues of self-confidence and esteem. For Debbie to be the support that she wants to be, but not over engaging.

Coaching supervisor: Thank you, Chris. Who else?

Kirsten: I'm really impressed at the level of self-reflection that Debbie is showing. And she seems to be thinking a lot and what it has to do with her and how she can respond in a great way to the client.

Svea: What I really appreciated is the way that Debbie talks about the interplay between what's happening between her and the client. She's given us glimpses into the client and herself, but also what's happening between them. What came to my mind was multifaceted, almost like light shining off different pieces. She described this young man, his life, the complexity and his future, but without getting overwhelmed with complicatedness.

Jane: I'm also a psychologist and a coach and what I really appreciated was Debbie is being mindful of the difference between therapy and coaching and explaining to that to the client. She wants to make sure she is being a coach.

Sukanya: I was impressed by the way Debbie has engaged with this young man. Because she doesn't know the number of sessions and it's about what the client wants. And every time so far he has said, there'll be a next session. I think it's the space that she creates, that safe space where he feels able to engage with her.

Cristina: I really appreciated the high desire of Debbie to deliver quality and to make sure that the client's experience is the one that matters. The other thing that was said at the end when she said, I want to make sure that I stay in the lane. Because I heard in there a lot around ethical aspects of coaching.

Stage 5: Reflecting

Coaching supervisor: Ok so we'll move into the final round. Take a moment to reflect on what you've heard. And something you might offer to Debbie for her to take away. This could be a story, an experience, a poem or an aphorism. Something that might be useful for her.

Jane: I heard that she's getting stuck. And I often find the clients where I'm stuck, I'm almost working

	harder than the client. It's about putting it back to the client and checking in with him. Is he seeing the progress that he wants? How would he know he doesn't need to come back? So having the endpoint in mind, what are they working towards but getting him to do that work? It's not for her to decide, but for asking him what he wants.
Svea:	What really stayed with me is this tender young man with the tattoos. And I wondered, how might they use this visual artistic imagery that he already has on his body as a way of tracking progress somehow? Is there something beyond all these words? And I wonder what tattoo he would give himself when he feels that this coaching has really helped him to become the business man that he would like to be. So the use of something visual not only wordy.
Coaching supervisor:	Thank you. Okay. Kirsten.
Kirsten:	I'm noticing, like, parallel processes here. So the young man wants advice from Debbie and Debbie wants advice from us to get unstuck. So I'm thinking, what would be some of the things have been useful from us and maybe using that to bring it back to her client.
Cristina:	Maybe it would be useful to go back and look at all of the ethical aspects of the relationship. How do you keep the boundaries clear? So I would say that would be an important aspect making clear that the coaching agreement is in there very straightforward and fixed and how the contracting was done. Just to make sure they need coaching.
Coaching supervision client:	I don't think I'm confused about the ethics anymore.

The coach may often want to comment on a suggestion which could lead to a longer dialogue between the coach and one of the team and take the process off track. So the aim of the supervisor here is to allow all members of the team to make suggestions first and then hand the space back to the coach to reflect on the suggestions.

Coaching supervisor:	Oh, hang on. I know you want to respond, but at this stage, just listen, and reflect on which of these ideas

	resonates best with you. Then you can respond what you'll take away. Okay. Who's next?
Chris:	One of the things that comes up for me, the story where Debbie shared and the young man was in tears because he hadn't had someone that believed in him. So my thought is what would be different if he could find people around him that really believed in him? Is that something that he has agency over? To look at who might be meaningful or impactful people in his life and what kind of a difference it would make if he were able to have more of their presence in his life.
Coaching supervisor:	Thank you. Any other thoughts?
Sukanya:	I'm thinking about how much you've been doing to get this young man to, think around how he responds to people around him. And this idea of wanting to be perfect and the fact that you are helping him to see criticism as an opportunity. And I wondered if you could help him work with that a bit more.

Stage 6: Closing

Coaching supervisor:	And so now I would invite Debbie what will you be taking away from today's session?
Coaching supervision client:	I'm almost moved to the point of tears. Each of you gave me a different perspective and a gift. So what I realised was this parallel learning that Kirsten raised, I realised that's exactly it. Just like my client wants affirmation, I need affirmation. And the parallel learning was. I struggle with perfectionism, just like this client. So I'm wanting to be exactly right as a coach. And I'm realising this is an important awareness that I bring. The idea of the ethics that Cristina raised has been a big red flag. And as she was speaking, things just clicked in my brain. And so I just felt compelled to say, well, no, it's not an issue anymore. But that was the result of this wonderful opportunity to reflect. Then I felt I was being very aware of the ethics and I stayed in the right lane. And then Svea raised this idea of how would you put a visual spin on how to contain or capture something that would be useful to the client. I'm going to use some of what Jane said

is I'm working too hard. I'm going to ask the client, supposing I gave you the right advice and you got what you needed, what would that look like? And what would that look like in the terms of what would be a visual memory. I really love what Chris said about this tender young man and the tears. And I have to admit we both cried because to hear someone say that they never had anything positive said to them was heartbreaking for me. So I felt like as a coach, that was the one thing I did right was to highlight that. I've also tried to remember Sukanya's idea. I think this has just been a lovely integration of what I need to do, which is to trust the client, trust to process and not be so hung up on my own performance. That's the takeaway. Thank you.

Coaching supervisor: Thank you, Debbie, I appreciate this reflecting team supervision process. It's always such a rich experience. Thank you all.

Index